QUIT SMOKING WITH CYTISINE

How to Stop Smoking Easily

By

Top Courses

TABLE OF CONTENTS

INTRODUCTION

Smoking habit (smoking) represents one of the most significant public health problems worldwide and is one of the significant risk factors for the development of neoplastic, cardiovascular, and respiratory diseases.

According to data from the World Health Organization, by 2030, smoking will cause 8 million deaths a year.

Contrary to conventional thinking, smoking is not responsible only for lung cancer, but also represents the leading risk factor for non-neoplastic respiratory diseases, such as chronic obstructive pulmonary disease (BPCO), and is one of the most important cardiovascular risk factors: smokers have a risk of mortality, due to coronary artery disease, 3 to 5 times higher than non-smokers.

Also, a person who smokes for life has a 50% chance of dying from a disease directly related to smoking, and his life may not exceed 45 to 54 years of age. In general, it goes considering that the quality of life of the smoker is severely compromised due to the higher frequency of respiratory (such as cough, phlegm, recurrent bronchitis, and asthma) and cardiac pathologies (such as hypertension, stroke and heart attack). For this reason, prevention initiatives implemented at the national and international levels are more and more. One of the first acts, dated 2004, was the "Who Framework Convention on Tobacco Control (Who Fctc)," the first international initiative to have expressed the need to control tobacco smoke for public health reasons. Numerous studies have consolidated the effectiveness of smoking bans on the trend of hospital admissions for acute myocardial infarction. Several studies have been conducted showing a reduction in critical coronary events between 2004 and the years following the introduction of the law, with values ranging from -4% to -13% of hospitalizations for heart attacks among people of working age. Addiction to nicotine contained in cigarettes constitutes the main obstacle to quitting smoking; however psychological and social factors also play an essential role. For this reason, there is no valid method for everyone. The period in which most smokers light their first cigarette is adolescence, when they try for the first time to "feel older", often under the influence of their companions. Educational interventions that involve school and family, privileged and more competent places to start educating on health and, specifically, preventing the habit of smoking are therefore fundamental. Data indicate that 90% of ex-smokers quit without help. If you can't stop on your own, the best thing to do is to hear from your GP and decide on a path together. It has been shown that the greater the support you receive, the higher the probability of quitting smoking permanently. Strategies for quitting smoking today include drug therapies and psychological support. This book is intended to be a support for those who decide to quit definitively through the conscious use of Citisina, a substance that, in recent years in Europe, has helped many people to eliminate cigarettes from their lives.

THE DEPENDENCE ON NICOTIN

The addiction to nicotine corresponds to the inability to stop taking this molecule, present in tobacco, despite the awareness that its intake is associated with serious health risks. Nicotine is a substance present in tobacco that can change the mood, triggering only temporarily pleasant sensations. Taking it can cause an addiction that makes it difficult to stop consuming tobacco despite being aware of the health problems associated with this habit. Tobacco smoke indeed contains more than 60 substances with a proven ability to cause cancer, as well as hundreds of other molecules harmful to health. Taken together, these substances damage almost all organs, so much so that more than 60% of people who do not quit smoking die from the consequences of this habit. The cause of addiction is nicotine's ability to increase neurotransmitter secretion involved in regulating mood and behavior. These include dopamine, a molecule involved in generating a feeling of pleasure. It is precisely this effect that generates addiction to tobacco. Symptoms of nicotine addiction include an inability to quit smoking, signs of withdrawal symptoms when trying to quit (anxiety, irritability, agitation, difficulty concentrating, bad mood, frustration, anger, increased appetite, insomnia, constipation or diarrhea), the inability to quit despite the fact that health problems have already appeared and prefer to smoke rather than agree to frequent environments (for example restaurants) where it is prohibited. The only way to avoid nicotine addiction is to never start smoking.

THE PHYSICAL DEPENDENCE

Although nicotine is in all respects an amazing substance, in small doses, it has many positive effects on the body. When taken in very small doses, nicotine slightly increases the heart rate, stimulates the metabolism, reduces the feeling of hunger, relieves stress and increases concentration. The problem arises when the nicotine dose increases. This substance is in fact extremely dangerous and the lethal dose for men is around 60mg taken through an injection directly into the vein. As soon as it is taken, nicotine spreads through the bloodstream and reaches the brain in seconds. Here, it stimulates the release of a substance called dopamine generating a sense of pleasure in the one who experiences it. At the same time, other important neurotransmitters are released, such as serotonin and adrenaline, which induce a feeling of euphoria in smokers. Physical addiction caused by nicotine it also depends on the need for our body to maintain high levels of dopamine and other substances. If an organism is used to taking a lot of nicotine, it will also require that a lot of dopamine is released. Conversely, those who smoke very little may not have the same need for dopamine as a hardened smoker. The brain's request for dopamine underlies both the addiction that nicotine causes in humans, but it is also the reason for the withdrawal symptoms that smokers experience when they try to quit. Failure to release dopamine causes the individual to be nervous, agitated and can also cause physical pain. Nicotine is a toxic substance, but it has never been proven that it is also carcinogenic. To completely detoxify from nicotine it takes an average of three weeks, but obviously this period of time can vary a lot from smoker to smoker. However, an ex-smoker will never be completely free from addiction from nicotine since our brain will always continue to request that pleasant release of dopamine and only your willpower will help you to quench the dopamine thirst of which your body is greedy. Technically it is possible to exceed the lethal dose of nicotine and cause an overdose, however the smoker will never get to such a point as our body has the ability to regulate itself. In short, sooner or later you will no longer want to continue smoking. Furthermore, combustion eliminates a part of the nicotine contained in tobacco. Much more dangerous are nicotine patches, if they are not used according to the indications on the package. Perhaps some of you will remember the scenes in the movie "thank you for smoking", where the protagonist is kidnapped and covered with nicotine patches thus risking a slow and painful death. The smoker who suffers from tobacco addiction cannot stop consuming the substance despite causing harm to your health. It is known that inhaled nicotine is a substance capable of inducing an addiction as strong as that established by heroin and cocaine. Tobacco users who start smoking as teenagers are usually more dependent on the substance than those who started as adults. Nicotine, a substance with psycho-active properties, causes craving for cigarettes, cigars, pipes, making smokers unable to easily quit and causing them physical and psychological symptoms when they abstain from smoking. While the nicotine contained in tobacco is addictive, the toxic effects are mainly due to other substances contained in tobacco smoke. Each cigarette quickly determines a decrease in the urgent need to smoke but desensitizes the nicotinic receptors and determines a consequent increase in their number, thus increasing the need for the next cigarette. This stimulation caused by the use of tobacco triggers chronic consumption. During the beginning phase of tobacco addiction, the smoker must increase the amount of nicotine administered in order to recreate the same intense sensations. After the first adaptation period, the smoker needs the individual dose of nicotine in order to regenerate the same intense sensations previously experienced. This morphological adaptation that occurs in the central nervous system corresponds to the development of a physical dependence. A person is considered to be addicted to nicotine when he has a history of chronic consumption with the following characteristics: substance abuse, continues to self-administer the substance despite the perceived adverse effects, records a high tolerance towards the substance and exhibits withdrawal symptoms when trying to quit. According to the criteria adopted by the World Health Organization

(WHO) in the International Classification of Diseases, tobacco addiction is included in: Mental and behavioral disorders due to tobacco use and has the disease code. Addiction syndromes refer to a set of physical, psychological, behavioral and cognitive phenomena, due to which the use of a substance (in this case tobacco) becomes a priority for the person concerned, disadvantaging other behaviors that in the past they had a higher value for that person.

How cigarettes are made up

Cigarettes are so familiar that we think we know the contents. In reality, it is a complex industrial product with countless variations that the smoker often ignores. Each cigarette is essentially made up of three elements. The most important is tobacco. Most cigarettes on the market contain a mixture of dried tobaccos that differ not only in the variety of the plant, but also in the manufacturing process: some are dried in dryers at controlled temperature and humidity, others in the sun, others are smoked. Cigarettes can also contain expanded and reconstituted tobacco: these are "reconstituted" tobacco processing waste in a foil through a physical and chemical process that involves the use of different substances such as carbon dioxide and freon. The second building block of cigarettes is paper: it is not simply a wrapper, but is used to regulate combustion and modify the characteristics of smoking. The important variable is its porosity: the more air can pass through the paper, the more the smoke compounds that pass through the cigarette are diluted. The last is the filter: the most common are made of cellulose acetate fibers glued together with a hardening agent (triacetin) which allows the filter to maintain its shape. But what are the additives contained in cigarettes? Just like food, cigarettes are also the result of an industrial process in which substances other than raw materials are used but essential to optimize the production process, improve product yield and meet customer tastes. Additives are the substances used for these purposes. Additives are used in the cigarette production process to facilitate the production process, for example by making seasoned tobacco less brittle. They fall into this group some compounds containing ammonia, carbon dioxide and ethyl alcohol. Some additives are used to aid combustion: among the substances used there are ammonium and sodium phosphate, sodium citrate and potassium citrate. Other additives instead serve to improve the flavor of cigarettes, both by introducing new notes and by masking the unpleasant ones. They range from licorice, to cocoa, from honey to fruit extracts and various spices. Then the additives are also used to: keep the tobacco moist and flexible, avoid the development of mold through preservatives, increase the mass of tobacco with the use of chemically inert substances, to optimize the release of nicotine for which compounds are used containing as ammonia. The combined use of these additives can also give secondary results: for example, the use of glycols not only makes the tobacco more flexible and promotes its conservation, but also ensures that the particles of smoke are held deeper in the lungs. The same applies to ammonia compounds: reacting with various tobacco compounds make the taste more acceptable. It is estimated that each cigarette contains at least 600 ingredients, which when burned create more than 7,000 different molecules. Of these, about 70 are now recognized as capable of causing cancer; for many others the ability to cause damage to health is known, so much so that their use is often regulated.

For example, here is a list of substances that are inhaled by smoking a cigarette, with the description of the uses for which they are known:

acetone: is a colorless and flammable liquid used as a solvent;

acetic acid: corrosive, can be irritating to the eyes, lungs and airways;

Stearic acid: found in nature in various types of fats, it is used, among other things, in the production of wax candles and in the cosmetic industry;

hydrogen cyanide: is one of the substances from which cyanide derives. It is used in chemical weapons, the Nazis who used it to produce the Zyklon B of the gas chambers also knew it;

acrolein: is a colorless, irritating and toxic liquid, also used in pesticide production;

aromatic amines: they are also used in the coloriating industries; carcinogens, are among the recognized risk factors for bladder cancers;

ammonia: is a colorless, toxic gas with a pungent smell. It also finds wide use in domestic use as a disinfectant;

Arsenic: is a highly toxic heavy metal, so much so that it is known from ancient times as poison;

benzene: is an aromatic hydrocarbon, also used as an additive for diesel and industrial solvents. It is carcinogenic;

butano: it is the same gas used in common lighters;

ethle chloride: is a chemical compound used as a component of PVC pipes;

esammine: is a chemical compound that is used as an ingredient for explosives;

formaldehyde: is an irritant for mucous and airways. It is also used in different household materials and products, it has been recognized as carcinogenic (causes nose-to-nose tumors and probably also leukaemia);

methanol , or methyl alcohol: it is used as areagent and industrial solvent, it is known as an illicit (and lethal) additive to sophistication wine;

naftalene: is a hydrocarbon obtained from the processing of tar, coal or oil. Its most well-known use is the production of anti-weapon

balls used in cupboards. It is suspected to be carcinogenic and damages red blood cells.
nitrous oxide (or **nitrogen monoxide):**also known as hilarious gas, it is used as an anesthetic and to boost the engines of racing cars;
Toluene: is an aromatic hydrocarbon used as a solvent, also in printing processes and paints, and as an antidetonant in the benzi-na; it has a harmful action on the nervous system, the kidneys, the eyes.

It is clear then ascertained the presence of:

mercury: it is a highly toxic, polluting and environmentally harmful heavy metal;
cadmium: is another heavy metal, among the most toxic components of batteries;
nichel: è un metallo contenuto in moltissimi materiali, cosmetici, alimenti; può provocare

irritazioni e dermatiti, nonché vere e pro- prie allergie.

Polonium 210 is a highly toxic element, with high radioactivity, and is actually among the substances present in smoking.

According to some studies, the main source of polonium 210 in smoking is presented by the fertilizers used in tobacco plantations, rich in polyphosphates containing radio, lead and polonium. Tobacco leaves accumulate these substances that over time gradually turn into polonium 210.

With the combustion of cigarettes the polonium reaches the bronchopulmonary apparatus, fixing mainly in the bifurcations of the smaller bronchi.

The presence of polonium 210 in cigarettes has been known since the 1960s, but it only became public knowledge in the 1980s.

HANDMADE CIGARETTES

What gives hand-rolled cigarettes more "naturalness" than packaged cigarettes is a false myth that probably arises from the idea that the harms of smoking are derived from the process of producing traditional cigarettes and not from the tobacco and its processing. In reality, tobacco used in rolled cigarettes undergoes production processes similar to those used in traditional cigarettes, although additives are used in different quantities and proportions to ensure the physical and taste characteristics of the rolled smoke. A recent New Zealand study, for example, showed that hand-rolled cigarettes contained at least 139 additives. The point in favour of rolled cigarettes is the lower amount of tobacco in them. However, often the smoker inhales more deeply to suck up the amount of nicotine he needs. This is probably why some studies have shown that hand-rolled cigarettes are more dangerous than traditional cigarettes.

LIGHT CIGARETTES

The light label refers in theory to the amount of harmful substances inhaled by the smoker. However, this is unreliable. Its measurement takes place with a machine (called a "smoking machine") that is not able to predict how the cigarette is consumed. It has been shown, for example, that the light cigarette smoker takes deeper puffs or covering the pores on the filter with his fingers, which would normally have the function of dispersing some of the inhaled substances. For these reasons many studies have shown that in cigarette smokers presented as light the dosage of toxic substances in the blood is not lower than that found in smokers of stronger cigarettes, nor does their risk of getting sick over time appear Reduced. Indeed, much research has shown a slightly higher risk of lung cancer in people who smoke light cigarettes. It also does not appear that the switch to light cigarettes reduces smoking addiction over time.

E-CIGARETTES

The electronic cigarette can be useful for controlling the nicotine addiction of smokers, because it allows you to avoid the tar and the many toxic gases contained in pipe smoke, cigars and cigarettes, exposing them to more limited risks. It is not yet clear whether it is effective as a quit smoking tool. Non-smokers should avoid electronic cigarettes, as nicotine promotes hypertension and diabetes (and in young people it can interfere with neurological development); furthermore, flavoring substances - also present in nicotine-free products - are suspected of exposing them to health risks. The name of electronic cigarette (often abbreviated in e-cig, from English) means a device that allows you to inhale steam, generally flavored, containing variable quantities of nicotine, which reaches the respiratory system without there being combustion of the tobacco and related harm. In smokers the practice of aspirating from the cigarette-shaped cylinder - for which the neologism "vaping" was coined - provides not only the nicotine that the organism that has developed dependence feels, but also a tactile, olfactory and gustatory experience that recalls that of the cigarette. The e-cig contain a variable amount of nicotine (generally, between 6 and 24 mg), in a mixture composed of water, propylene glycol, glycerol and other substances, including flavoring. Some models do not contain nicotine, but only a flavored vapor. The principle was developed for the first time in China, and this type of device had its first significant diffusion also in the West around 2006. According to the 2016 Annual Report on Smoking of the Higher Institute of Health, today about two million Italians make occasional or regular use of electronic cigarettes. On the market there are numerous devices that have different shapes, but have three elements in common: the inhaler (the so-called cartridge, which contains the liquid substance to be sprayed); an atomizer (the element that heats and vaporizes the liquid); the battery that powers the atomizer. The amount of nicotine taken can be adjusted according to individual needs. Several studies have reported the presence of potentially harmful substances in the vapor produced by electronic cigarettes. Propylene glycol has been used for some time, for example in smoke bombs used in the film industry and in pop concerts, and is generally considered safe, although some studies indicate that prolonged inhalation may give rise to airway irritation, coughing and in very rare cases asthma and rhinitis. Among other things, the heating of propylene glycol and glycerin can produce formaldehyde and acetaldehyde, both of which are carcinogenic potential, even if the quantities associated with the consumption of e-cig appear modest. Even on the complete safety of the substances used to flavor the aerosol, certainties are lacking. For example the diacetyl, an aroma widely used among other things in butter, it is safe when it is ingested, but it is associated with the onset of obliterating bronchiolitis if it is inhaled for long periods in high concentrations. According to a study published in April 2017 in a journal of the American Society of Physiology, there are about 7,000 different flavoring compounds contained in electronic cigarettes for sale in the United States, with highly variable biochemical characteristics. In light of the preliminary tests carried out, the researchers conclude that these compounds "should be examined one by one in depth to determine the potential toxicity in the lung or elsewhere". Among the possible dangers associated with the use of electronic cigarettes, it should not be forgotten that linked to poisoning by accidental contact with the nicotine-based liquid contained in the cartridges, possible if the electronic cigarette is used when lying down. In recent years they have increased reports to poison control centers related to the intoxication of young children, which according to a study published in Pediatrics in 2016, have also gone from one per month in 2010 to 223 per month in 2015 in the United States. Overall, despite the need for further studies, the consensus is now wide that in comparison with traditional consumption of tobacco products, electronic cigarettes ensure a significant reduction in damage for the smoker and for those who live next to him (there do not seem to be effects similar to those of passive smoking) . A study published in February 2017 in the Annals of Internal Medicine (funded by Cancer Research UK) has confirmed for the first time that abandoning the traditional cigarette for the benefit of the electronic cigarette leads to a significant reduction in substances after only six months carcinogens present in the body. However, compared to the initial reassurances of the producers on the total harmlessness of electronic cigarettes and their effectiveness as a tool to overcome nicotine addiction, some question marks remain that require further research. A systematic review of all the studies in the scientific literature, published in the journal Lancet Respiratory Medicine, caused a sensation in 2016, since it concluded that even the use of the electronic cigarette by smokers - who do not always use it with the aim of quit - would be associated with a lower chance of defeating nicotine addiction.

A BRIEF CHRONICLE OF THE USE OF CYTISINE

Quitting smoking is possible, you have to clear the battlefield of obstacles killing motivation: beliefs, advice of the friend on duty. You have to have solid weapons and shun DIY. The most effective therapy, according to international medicine, is the integrated psychomotive and behavioral counseling therapy with one or more first-line drugs. Alongside the traditional nicotinic substitutes, Bupropione and Vareniclina, the tuxedo cessation landscape is now joined by a new one: Citisina. The flowers of the plant from which this molecule is extracted, Cytisus Laburnum, vulgarly known as Maggiociondolo, are yellow and seemingly harmless, can hang in clusters in pretty ornamental canopies. However, The Majority, beyond its inoffensive appearance, is well known in the Anti-Poison Centers. Yet it is a plant that cures: numerous studies show that Citisine derived from Maggiociondolo is a valuable help to quit smoking. The toxicity of Cytisine depends on the dosage. Like nicotine, Cytisine is toxic if ingested in large quantities. Therefore, if one of the first cases of human intoxication of Cytisine, due to ingestion of the seeds of the plant, was documented in 1878 by Wiegand, in Europe traditional medicine recommended alcohol extracts containing Cytisine for constipation, migraine, insomnia, cough and neuralgia and about 100 years ago, Cytisina was used as an asthmatic, antisivesis and acid. Extracts are used in homeopathy against air sickness, migraines and nervous insomnia, and in stress from mental overwork. In the past the most widespread use was diuretic use. Recently anti-inflammatory and hypoglycemic properties have been attributed to Citisina But the virtue of the molecule is found above all in the fight against smoking. Citisine has been used since 1960 in Eastern Europe for the cessation of smoking. But the news of use in this field, albeit empirically, goes back two decades: Russian soldiers during World War II smoked Cytisus Laburnum leaves to replace tobacco, which is difficult to find. The first clinical study on Citisina in tuxedo cessation was carried out by Stoyanov and Yanachkova in 1965. In recent decades, at least a dozen pharmacological and clinical studies have been produced, mainly in Eastern European countries, demonstrating the good efficacy and safety of the Citisine-based drug. Currently the drug can be bought freely under the name Tabex in Poland and Russia and on prescription in the other countries of the former Soviet Union. Tabex, which seems to bode well, is now widespread in 20 regions: in Poland alone in 2013 it reported the sale of about 600,000 packages. An important factor that has led to its widespread spread, especially in the East, is its low cost compared to Bupropione and Vareniclina. Cytisine is highly effective and costs about a tenth less than other drug therapies. This is why Citisin is much more competitive than other smoking drugs. The treatment schemes used so far involve short pathways, about 25 days with the drug starting at the maximum dosage, 6 tablets per day, and then a scaling. In this scheme, Cytisine is taken orally in tablets (1.5 mg of cytisine per tablet) for 25 days: starting from one tablet every 2 hours, with progressive reduction to one tablet every six hours. Users are advised to reduce the number of cigarettes they smoke in the first five days of treatment, with a recommended "stop smoking" date on the fifth day. Citisine is therefore an opportunity with an excellent cost-benefit ratio for smokers who want to quit.

STOP WITH CYTISINE

Cytisine is a molecule known since the early 1960s for the treatment of smoking. It is an alkaloid found in Cytisus laburnum, which behaves like a partial agonist of nicotine receptors. The first studies were conducted in Eastern European countries and showed a good profile of effectiveness, but nevertheless the commercialisation of the drug in Western countries was limited by European legislation. Pharmacological studies indicate a short half-life of the substance, which is eliminated for 90-95% by kidney. Recently, several clinical trials have brought attention to cytisine, which has shown superior smoking cessation effectiveness compared to both placebo and nicotine, between 8% (at 12 months) and 22% at 6 months, depending on the studies. The most reported adverse events consist of disorders of the digestive system (nausea, dyspepsia, dry mouth), insomnia, drowsiness or headache. A significant factor is the relatively low cost of the drug. In 2014, the NHS produced a paper assessing the cost of drug treatments of smoking, concluding that cytisine has the most favourable profile among the drugs considered.

WHAT IS CYTISINE

Knowing **what cytisine is** can help those who plan to quit smoking but fail to do so, to make one last attempt. This substance seems to be particularly effective in the fight against nicotine addiction, which is responsible for tobacco addiction. Pharmaceutical experts consider it to be the aspirin of the fight against smoking: yet it is a molecule that has been rediscovered for some time. In fact, the discovery of cytisine dates back to the 1960s and has always had excellent effects in the fight against dependence on cigarette smoking.

Initially the use was limited to a few countries, but later the entire West was able to discover the great **potential** of this molecule. The effectiveness of cytisine has also been attested through studies published in leading scientific journals.

Many wonder what cytisine is and how it manages to explain its **benevolent action** in the body. It is important to know, first of all, that cytisine is a molecule of plant origin extracted from Mayciondolo which is a plant very similar to tobacco. Its mechanism of action can be explained precisely because of its similarity to the structure of nicotine. Just like the main substance of tobacco, cytisine also acts on a **nicotinic receptor.** When the action of that receptor is blocked by cytisine, nicotine cannot go to have any action on the same receptor. The result is the reduction or even complete elimination of the sense of gratification that is induced by cigarette smoking. This is why withdrawal symptoms are significantly reduced and, above all, the desire to light a cigarette is also reduced.

Data on cytisine-based treatments to overcome **nicotine addiction** were extremely positive. In fact, according to studies in New Zealand, as many as 40% of cytisine-treated smokers actually managed to quit smoking. A better effectiveness than that of nicotine which is 31%. This opens up new therapeutic perspectives that focus on what cytisine is. It should be remembered, however, that cytisine can be purchased in the pharmacy only after presentation of a prescription for masterful gallenic preparation, that is, made directly in the pharmacy.

Importantly, the effect of cytisine can be affected by concomitant therapy with antitubercular drugs.

In any case, it is always good to inform your doctor if you are taking or have recently taken medications of any kind, including prescription medicines and herbal products.

Cytisine, although it is a well-tolerated drug, should be given with great caution in patients suffering from certain types of pathologies, such as:

Surrene cancer;

Schizofrenia;

Chronic heart failure;

Hyperthyroidism;

Diabetes mellitus;

Cerebrovascular pathologies;

Gastroesophageal reflux;

Peptic ulcer and/or duodenal ulcer in remission;

Kidney and/or liver failure.

In addition, cytisine should also be given with caution in patients under 18 years of age and in elderly patients over 65 years of age.

Cytisine is usually well tolerated at therapeutic doses, but can still cause side effects, although not all patients manifest them. The main side effects that have been reported as a result of the use of high doses of cytisine include:

Headaches;

Heartburn;

Nausea;

Vomiting;

Digestive disorders;

Dizziness;

Muscle weakness;

Tachycardia.

Cytisine is available for oral administration in the form of capsules. The capsules must be taken whole, without chewing, with the help of a glass of water. Cytisine treatment has a duration of 25 days and it is necessary to stop smoking by the fifth day of therapy. Generally, in the first three days of treatment, you start with taking 1.5 mg of the drug six times a day. Subsequently, the daily dose of medication will be gradually decreased according to a precise posoological pattern, until you get to the last days of therapy in which you will take 1.5 mg of cytisine once or twice a day. In any case, the doctor may decide to vary the posology depending on the patient's response to therapy.

Therefore, it is essential to always follow the directions given by the doctor, both in terms of the amount of medication to be taken, and with regard to the frequency of administration and the duration of treatment.
Due to the possible damage it could cause in the fetus or baby, the use of cytisine by pregnant women and by breastfeeding mothers is not recommended.
It is recommended that those who decideto use cytisine as a smoking remedy contact their doctor to define possible problems related to its use.
It is absolutely necessary to consult a doctor to define the right daily posology according to the number of cigarettes smoked now and on the basis of one's physical state.
It is not possible to self-heal with this type of method, because in addition to risking relapse, the clinical picture of the patient must be evaluated in advance.

Preliminaries: Patient Assessment

To achieve higher rates of cessation of tobacco use, all smokers must be systematically identified during each medical examination, regardless of whether the patient is being treated for a tobacco-related disease. For this purpose, the best opportunities are occasional or annual medical examinations, as most citizens visit their doctor at least once a year, or regularly/occasionally meet a dentist, other specialist doctor or health professional for health reasons or other reasons. All doctors, regardless of their specialty, should use these occasions to identify smokers and arrange therapy to cease consumption. Clinical evaluation of tobacco consumption is a necessary medical act and must be legitimized as a routine intervention. Smoking status and tobacco consumption, as recommended by these guidelines for the cessation of tobacco consumption, must be recorded in patients' health records: such as hospital admission or discharge documents, submissions to other facilities, laboratory analysis reports, etc.

The type of tobacco product consumed gives us an idea about the level of addiction, as nicotine dependence is more severe in cigarette users, than those using cigars, pipes, steam pipes, e-cigarettes or oral tobacco.

Tobacco consumption can be defined as:

Number of cigarettes smoked per day;

Number of cigarette packets/ann

Then we have to make ananalysis of previous attempts to quit smoking.

The experience of previous cessation attempts has been shown to be highly predictive of future quitting attempts and can be used to guide future treatment.

It is recommended to explore in the medical evaluation:

It is the number of past cessation attempts,

It's the longest period of abstinence from smoking,

Any previous cessation treatment and what the treatment consisted of,

It's any history of withdrawal symptoms,

Any risk factors for relapses,

Positive aspects described during abstinence.

These characteristics are important for calculating the probability of success of treatment or its failure, as well as compliance with the treatment and the patient's ability to overcome the withdrawal crisis.

Then understand what the patient's motivation is for the cessationof cigarette use.

It is recommended to evaluate the motivation of a smoker in quitting smoking. All doctors should evaluate the motivation of their smoking patients. There are various methods that can be used to assess the motivation in quitting smoking, which are described here.

The reasoning can be assessed through direct questions, including:

Do you want to quit smoking (now)?

If you decide to quit smoking, how sure are you to be successful?

What are the reasons why you want to give up smoking?

How important is it for you to quit smoking?

Some doctors then de-escalate a laboratory dignosis of tobaccoaddiction.

Smoking status as defined by clinical criteria can also be assessed by biochemical tests for the evaluation of biomarkers of tobacco smoke exposure, such as the concentration of carbon monoxide in the breathed air and the level of cotinine (a nicotine metabolite).

Carbon monoxide measurement is often used as a tool to increase the patient's motivation to quit. The fast conversion of carbon monoxide to normal values encourages the smoker to be abstinent and therefore, by showing lower carbon monoxide values at each control visit, the attempt toquit is supported. It is true, however, that there is insufficient evidence to support the use of carbon monoxide control over standard treatment. Because of its value as a motivational tool, specialized smoking cessation centers should be equipped with a carbon monoxide analyzer.

Cotinine is the main metabolite of nicotine and is a biomarker of exposure to tobacco smoke. By monitoring the concentration of cotinine in the body, exposure to an individual's smoke can be assessed. Cotinine can be measured in blood, hair, saliva and urine. The lifetime of nicotine is about two hours; however the nicotine concentration can vary depending on the time of day the last cigarette was smoked. Cotinine has a lifetime of 15-20 hours and as such can be used to measure withdrawal from smoking in the last 24-48 hours.

PRELIMINATORS: IDENTIFY THE MOTIVATION

Motivation is essential for any smoker who wants to quit. Therefore, methods to strengthen the patient's motivation are particularly important in smoking cessation practices

As for the operator:

The operator must show a clear interest in trying to understand the patient. To make this interest concrete, it is good to make reflections and summaries on what the patient said during the interview.

The operator must help the patient, given his goals and values, to become aware of the gap between the current and future situation. Being aware of wide discrepancies between how we are and how we would like to be is crucial in initiating possible behavioral changes.

Patient resistances must be respected and seen as a natural sign of anxiety and doubts about change. If the operator confronts or argues with the patient, his resistance increases. It is more useful to try to circumvent resistance while trying to prevent conflict situations during the interview.

The operator supports the patient's self-esteem by showing confidence in his abilities of change and expressing appreciation for the efforts made during the termination practices.

As for the patient, the discourse is a little more complex. There are many questions that those who decide to quit smoking ask themselves.

The relationship with smoking is in fact strong, complex, intimate. And maturing the decision to quit is difficult as it happens in some relationships that you do not want to give up, even it has long been understood that they do more harm than good. In order to be able to choose a smoke-free life once and for all, it is necessary to overcome the psychological traps that lead us to believe that, after all, the pleasure that is taken from each cigarette is greater than the risks that are taken. It is important to be aware that the dangers of smoking are not abstract numbers, but that the statistics affect each smoker personally. You have to work on your self-esteem and convince yourself of the ability to do it. And at the same time you must not be afraid or ashamed to ask for help.

Patient Q&A to Find Motivation

I'm reducing the number of cigarettes smoked. What's the need to stop?

It is true that quantitycan makea difference, in terms of health risks, and that the less you smoke thebetter,the more true it is that no cigarette is risk-free.
Clinical data show that smoking even as little as five days a monthcan lead to coughing and breathlessness, and that smoking less than four cigarettes a day can also increase the risk of death from heart attack and other diseases. Even with such a small number of cigarettes smoked, the risk of cancer and respiratory diseases remains higher than average. Like smoked cigarettes (even a few), the risk seems

to be greater for women than for men, especially for lung cancer.
So even for those who smoke so little thatthey hesitate to call themselves smokers, there are good reasons to quit altogether. Taking into account that there is an extra weapon:compared to heavy smokers, those who smoke little have a lower nicotine-dependentness, and therefore an easier-to-break bond.

Smoking helps me manage stress. I don't think I can do without it.

One of the great deceptions of smoking is one that led people to think that cigarettes help manage stress. In reality,it is the desire to smoke that makes you feel stressed and anxious; feelings that are relieved when you smoke a cigarette, in virtue of a vicious circle.

The reasons for this phenomenon are all in nicotine, a real drug that causes addiction. Nicotine acts on a large number of mechanisms in the brain: for example, it stimulates the release of dopamine, a substance that has among its effects to produce a feeling of good-naturedness. In smokers, cigarettes become a triggering mechanism for the production and release of these substances, so as addiction grows, the need to enjoy its effects grows. From these mechanisms arises the need to smoke, which for the smoker is a condition of constant stress that only subsides when he lights a cigarette. However, this is a temporary benefit: as concentration in the body decreases, the mechanism is set in motion again, raising stress levels.

This is why, on average, smokers have higher levels of stress than those who do not smoke. The good news is that after three months of abstinence from smoking the body stops needing the stimulus from nicotine, and the control of these mechanisms by the body returns to a normal state.

I've been smoking for so many years. What's the point of quitting now?

It is true: the longer you smoked, the more damage cigarettes have already caused to the body. However it is important to keep in mind that at any age (andeven if you smoke for many years) it is always worth quitting.
Leaving the cigarette has both long-term and immediate effects.
A smoker who quit smoking at 50 halves the risk of dying in the next 15 years. At 65, he has a risk of dying comparable to those who have never smoked. In addition, even at an older age quitting smoking reduces the risk of going to heart disease and cancer. Overall, for those who are older with the years and have a longer

experience with cigarettes, it is also the immediate effects that are worth quitting for: the improvement of circulation and the ability to breathe, with the greater energy that It has a tangible impact on quality of life at a time when any physical limitation risks anticipating the loss of self-sufficiency.

I've already stopped smoking before, but I've always recovered. Is it worth a try again?

Sure. And past experience can be of great use to succeed in effectively quitting, once and for all. Before trying to quit smoking again it is good to have a plan and above all analyze why in the past you have not managed to achieve the goal. Understanding what they helped and which have led to rekindling the cigarette may be the first step in abandoning the habit of smoking once and for all.

I'm convincing myself that it's better to quit smoking. But I'm looking for the good opportunity to do it

It is a common condition for many smokers to look for an opportunity that motivates to quit smoking. But just think about it for a moment to realize that life is full of good opportunities. The first of the year, for example. Who doesn't make good New Year's resolutions? Starting the year by losing the bad habit of smoking is one of the most beautiful gifts you can give yourself. It's also convenient: to count the days and then the weeks and months since you left the cigarette just look at the calendar.
Or when spring approaches: it's time when many start thinking about getting fit for summer. Adopt a healthier diet and start exercising regularly fit perfectly with the choice to say goodbye to cigarettes. It will gain its health, and it will also gain its appearance:

smoking, in fact, makes the skin dull and dull. It also makes you look more tired and lacking in energy.

Quitting by spring, then, can be really decisive for allergy sufferers who at this time of year give maximum symptoms, which worsen further if you smoke.

In summer you can take the opportunity of the beginning of the holidays, or do it for mountain walks or swims to the sea that will be less difficult if you do not smoke. And so on: scrolling through the calendar there is no month when you can not find a good reason to smoke.

Not to mention the great occasions of life. When you want to have a child, since smoking affects fertility, or the moment you become a parent or grandfather, and the additional motivation to quit may be protecting the child from passive smoking, or simply the desire to increase the chances of seeing it grow for many years. Or when changing jobs: several studies show that superiors tend to see with a better eye the employees who do not smoke. The occasions, in short, are not lacking, bauctionseize them, or more simply find their own.

I'd like to stop but it's not the right time.

It is true: not all times are as suitable for quitting smoking. In particularly stressful times trying to give up the cigarette can turn out to be a boomerang: you risk not having the strength to cut to smoke, and thereby compromising the motivation to quit.
So it is good to choose wisely the time to engage, assessing whether in that period there are particular external factors that can influence its success. The important thing is that the search for the right moment does not become an excuse to postpone it, and that once

the decision to stop is made, it is pursued to the full.

I'd like to quit but I guess I can't. I'm too addicted.

Nicotine addiction is not easy to beat and is all the stronger the longer and more intensely you have smoked. There is no doubt about that, but just think that every year tens of thousands of people stop smoking to understand that it is possible to do it.

You need to have a good deal of determination, and the ideal is to get help from a professional. To fear not to make it and to be aware of one's addiction is neither an evil nor a sign of weakness. On the contrary: it is a first step to put in perspective your relationship with smoking and to prepare for the inevitable symptoms of abstinence, such as irritation, fatigue, poor concentration.

I'd like to quit smoking. But I don't want to gain weight.

It's true, almost all people who stop smoking gain weight. However, it is important to know that there is no automation: if and how much you will get fat depends more on how you behave when you leave the cigarette than on the effects of smoking.
On average, those who quit smoking weigh between 4 and 5 kilos in weight within the first few weeks. About 30 percent of this increase (1.5 kg, on average) comes from the loss of the direct effects of the cigarette on the body, especially those on basal metabolism that leads it to consume more calories. The remaining fattening is related to the fact that one tends to feel the appetite more. Often much of this weight gain comes from out-of-hours snacks that tend to compensate for the lack of cigarettes, with the gestures associated with it.

In many cases, therefore, the decision to choose for daily snacks calorie-poor foods (such as fruits and vegetables) can alone greatly reduce the additional calorie intake, and with it weight gain. If you could take the opportunity to exercise regularly (it takes thirty minutes a day of sustained walking) you could even avoid weight gain or even limit it further.

In any case, even without these precautions, several studies show that the extra kilos taken during the period when smoking stopped are in many cases disposed of in the first year by non-smokers. It is therefore good to focus on your goal and keep in mind that those few kilos will be disposed of calmly and that the benefits of stopping smoking far outweigh the damage of weight gain.

I've decided to quit. How likely are I to make it?

It is good to know from the start: quitting smoking is not easy, and the risks of failure are quite high. Nicotine addiction is very strong and stopping intake can produce symptoms that, at least in the very first few days, can have a strong impact on daily life. In addition, even when the symptoms disappear the need to smoke can recur. The chances of doing so vary greatly from person to person: but three factors seem more than others to influence the chances of success:

how long it has been smoked;

the number of cigarettes smoked daily;

the extent of withdrawal symptoms that you experience when trying to quit.

In general, women seem to be more likely to fail. The reasons are still to be clarified, but it is likely that it is likely that for a woman it is more complicated to get out of addiction for psychological and physiological reasons: it is more difficult to give up a social attitude, gesture, it is more feared the fallout on mood and social pressures.

QUIT DAY

In all tobacco cessation pathways, quit day is provided, that is, the day when you stop smoking permanently. This day is often seen with fear and anxiety, a kind of day of "universal judgment", the ordeal through which the smoker must pass to purify himself. Nomore wrong. The quit day should be seen with the trepidation of the last day of school or the last day of work before the holidays. Not the day you face an exam, but the day you experience a change. For the better.

But how to manage this day?
The quit day must be experienced from the day before! The previous day it is advisable to throw lighters, advanced cigarette packets, ashtrays and anything that might remind you of the cigarette. It is also appropriate to eliminate everything that, smelling of smoke, could

trigger the urge to smoke: wash the car, take a nice shower and wash your hair, prepare clean clothes to wear the next day (from underwear to coat). Warn relatives, friends, colleagues: "Tomorrow I stop smoking, don't offer me cigarettes."

What to do on quit day?

The first rule is: change habits. Some suggestions:1. If you have been prescribed medications, take them according to the prescribed posology. It has been studied in anticipation of this day, do not increase it because you need a "reinforcement." If you have breakfast at home in the morning, go to the bar (and vice versa)3. put chewing gum and/or candy in your pocket (sugar free) to use during the day4. Bring a pen, a keychain, a cocoa butter or lipstick, or any other small object to fiddle with when you're on break or don't have your hands full.5. move to another time the "coffee break" or better notto drink coffee!! 6. Take a bottle of water to drink immediately after the coffee (if you just can't make it to meno), in place ofthe cigarette. Remember: do not counteract the urge to smoke. It lasts a few minutes so use the "trick" of the water bottle whenever you feel the need. It works!7. If you always have lunch in the same place, go home or eat at the office or change premises8. When you are in company, tell everyone that you have stopped smoking: make sure that they do not offer you cigarettes and do not smoke in your presence or near you. Don't try to "not think about cigarettes" otherwise you'll just think about them all day. But in case the thought assaults you and it's too annoying, stand up and do something. Anything: Take a walk, take out the trash, retune the decoder, no matter what you do, as long as you're active.

One last tip: don't load your quit day with too many meanings. It is not the beginning of a new life, the world in general (and yours in particular) will not become more beautiful: the work will always be stressful, the mortgage installments will always be the same, your neighbor will always keep the television volume too high and your favorite team will lose the derby for yet another volta. You will only find that you can deal with all this even without cigarettes.

For restor, well also remember these benefits: "After 20 minutes the blood pressure and heart rate return to normal " After 24 hours the lungs begin to cleanse from mucus and deposits left by smoking, the halitosis improves. Improve taste and smell" After 3 days you start to breathe better and you recover energy " After 2-12 weeks the blood circulation improves" After 3-9 months the improvement in breathing is more marked. Coughs and hisses disappear or subside." After 1 year, cardiovascular risk has halved compared to that of those who continue to smoke. the oesophagus and bladder have halved after 10 years the risk of lung cancer in many cases has returned equal to that of those who have never smoked or in any case halved (this depends on many factors: the number of cigarettes smoked daily, the number of years in which you have smoked, any concurrent pathologies etc.) After 15 years the risk of heart disease (e.g. heart attack) at the same level as for non-smokers. Mortality (for all causes taken into account) reaches almost the same level as people who have never smoked.

THE STATUS OF CURRENT STUDIES IN U.S.A.

The National Center for Complementary and Integrative Health (NCCIH), a section of the U.S. government's National Institutes of Health (NIH), has promoted research into the therapeutic use of Cytissina as a natural smoking cessation drug. The aim of the research is to produce the necessary scientific documentation for the Food and Drug Administration (FDA) approval process. The study is funded through a partnership between public and private bodies involving some NIH institutions and centres, industrial partners and industry consultants.

Citisina, in order to enter the U.S. market as a smoking cessation treatment substance, requires FDA approval based on clinical trials. The NCCIH project aims to provide the FDA with the scientific investigation necessary to put Citisine on the list of substances allowed for anti-smoking therapies.

OTHER RESEARCH ON CITISINE

Cytisine is a partial agonist of the nicotinic receptor substance isolated over 50 years ago from the Cytisus laburnum plant. In some Eastern European countries, Cytisine has been used for several decades as a useful substance in anti-smoking therapies. Over these years, scientific studies and clinical trials have been conducted such as those published in the New England Journal of Medicine in 2011 and 2014:

In the first study entitled Placebo-controlled trial of cytisine for tuxedo cessation,conducted in Poland, Cytisine proved to be more effective than placebo;

In the second study entitled "Cytisine versus nicotine for tuxedo cessation", conducted in New Zealand, Citisina was found to be more effective than nicotine replacement therapy.

Despite the evidence, scientific studies conducted so far on Citisina have not been considered definitive or sufficient by the US authorities to approve its use in smoking cessation therapies.

Clinical studies Stoyanov S. and M. Yanachkova studied the use of Citisina in 70 volunteers with long experience as smokers and observed that 57% had managed to quit smoking, while in 31.4% of cases a partial result was obtained, i.e. a reduced cigarettes from 20-30 to 3-4 per day. The results were negative in 11% of patients, following premature abandonment of therapy, that is, before the third day of treatment (the period of time required to saturate the body). In a second group of 17 smokers with serious mental illnesses (schizophrenia, epilepsy and reactive psychosis), the administration of Cytisine together with neuroleptics, antidepressants and insulin led 5 patients to quit smoking and induced a decrease 7 others. Cytisine did not interact negatively with other medications taken by patients.

Vlaev S. et al. considered the possibility of controlling depressive symptoms in 5 patients with psychogenic and periodic depression, in parallel with the treatment of pathological desire to smoke. Cytisine was administered in gradually increasing doses up to a maximum daily dose of 15 mg (5 tablets 3 times a day). The authors observed a rapid reduction in depressive symptoms, achieving improvement in patients with reactive depression as early as the end of the first week and by the end of the second week in patients with periodic depression. Side effects included a slight muscle tension and an equally slight decrease in blood pressure. The antidepressant action of the drug is explained by the increase in the level of cateculamine, especially that of adrenaline, which is generally reduced in depressed patients.

Paun D. and J. Franze of Friedrichscheim Hospital in Berlin studied the therapeutic efficacy of Cytisine in 266 smokers, comparing it with the effect in 239 placebo-treated patients. Therapeutic results were compared to the 4th, 8th, 13th and 26th week of treatment. Patients with a serious intention to quit smoking had priority. By the 8th week, 55% of patients treated with Citisina had quit smoking, which was reduced to 21% at the end of the 26th week. However, recurrences in the main group still reduced the average number of smoked cigarettes to half. The authors point out that the effect in the group treated with Citisine compared to the placebo-treated group is statistically significant and conclude that the drug can be used successfully when the patient has a serious intention to quit smoking.

Experts also treated 366 smokers with concomitant bronchitis with Cytisina compared to 239 placebo-treated patients. After completing the treatment cycle (of a maximum duration of 4 weeks), 55% of patients stopped smoking, while in the placebo group there was an effect in only 34%. Of the 230 smokers with chronic bronchitis treated with Cytisine, 85% stopped smoking by the end of the 4th week, 66% after 8 weeks and after 23 weeks 46%. Almost all patients who had quit smoking showed a subjective improvement in bronchitic symptoms.

F. Schmidt conducted a test for the use of 14 different substances out of 1975 smokers using a double-blind placebo-controlled experiment.

Cytisine was given to 181 patients. Results show that patients treated with Citisine had the optimal improvement, in fact in the group treated with Citisina 103 patients (57%) quit smoking, while after 3 months this percentage dropped to 38%. Cytisine is followed by the drugs Ni-Perlen (54% and 48% respectively), Atabakko (54% and 29%, respectively), both nicotine substitutes, Citotal (lobelina sulfate, 50% and 36%, respectively), unilobin, potassium chloride, potassium granule, citrate of potassium, nicobrevin, targophagin, etc. Volunteers had received instructions in the mail regarding how to treat them, thus avoiding the influence of extra-pharmacological factors, so the results recorded by the patients themselves in the application forms are extremely reliable.

West and Zatonsky resumed studies on Citisine, which were adapted to the standards required by modern research. In 2004 it was found that Citisina had, in the long term, an efficacy comparable to nicotine substitutes. In an uncontrolled 2006 study, 14% of subjects treated with Citisina were still abstinent at 12 months, while a study vs. Citisina was still in a 12-month study. placebo published in 2011 in NEJM showed an 8.4% percentage of patients still abstinent after one year. Based on the most relevant multicentric clinical-pharmacological studies, the following general conclusions regarding the therapeutic efficacy of Cytisine can be drawn: The drug has been tested on 1045 volunteers, compared to 400 patients treated with 1500 patients treated with other anti-smoking drugs. Results show that 55-76% of patients treated with Cytisine quit smoking. These percentages, derived from several studies, are statistically significant and are higher than those of other substances compared. Cytisine has shown a good effect on chronic lung diseases associated with prolonged smoking, as well as on patients with mental illnesses of a depressive nature. No serious side effects have been reported, if warnings and contraindications (severe hypertension and atherosclerosis) are observed. An improvement in the general state of patients has been observed due to the suspension of chronic nicotine intoxication. An active approach is needed towards patients who have failed the first treatment, causing them to repeat the cycle with an interval of 4-5 months. In a very recent study, placebo controlled, (Walker et al 2014) and conducted in New Zealand on more than 1300 patients, Citisin was significantly superior to nicotine in the treatment of smoke deprivation. Up to 1 month of continuous abstinence from smoking was found for 40% of participants who used Cytisina, but only 31% in "replacement" nicotine recipients, for a difference of 9.3

percentage points (95% confidence interval, 4.2-14.5). Citisine's effectiveness in continued abstinence was found to be higher than nicotine treatment at 1 week, 2 months and 6 months, both among men and women.

WHEN YOU CAN DEFINE YOURSELF AS TOBACCO-FREE

The first positive effects on the body are already 20 minutes after it has stopped. But improvements and changes occur as the days pass, although it can take up to 9 months to completely free the body from nicotine, and to significantly lower the risk of cancer takes ten years.

After 20 minutes

It seems little, but already after 20 minutes something changes in the body: blood pressure stabilizes and improves, pulses drop and heart rate normalizes.

After 8 hours

Psychologically it is a very difficult time, but the physique is already benefiting from the choice: the levels of carbon monoxide in the blood drop (in cigarettes there are high concentrated nicotine, carbon monoxide and tar), oxygen levels return to normal while nicotine decreases to more than 93 percent

After 24 hours

It is the peak of the intensity of symptoms from nicotine deficiency, such as depression, irritability, frustration, anxiety. But it pays off by the return to normality of carbon monoxide levels

After 48 hours

It's been two days and things are starting to get better, especially with regard to the sense of taste and smell, which are recovered by donating skills and sensitivities that seemed forgotten

After 72 hours

On the third day it is the breath that benefits from the choice to quit smoking, especially if under strain. However, desire increases, and many people have reported seeing flu-like symptoms, insomnia, difficulty resting, changes in appetite, dizziness

Between 2 weeks and 9 months later

Negative side effects disappear: blood circulation improves, lung work normalizes, smoker's coughs disappear and nasal congestion, walking becomes easier and physical energy increases, as well as the sense of fatigue and exhaustion. But above all, it's the time when the whole copro gets rid of the presence of nicotine

After 1 year

Heart and arteries show the greatest improvement: risk of coronary heart disease, myocardial infar heart attack and stroke drops by 50 percent

After 5 years

The risk of brain hemorrhage (ESA) drops by 41 percent, while the risk of stroke is equal to the levels of those who have never smoked. For women ex-smokers, the threat of getting diabetes drops to the level of women who have never smoked

After 10 years

Even for men the danger of getting diabetes drops to non-smoking levels. The best news is the risks of cancers: the risk of cancer drops to the mouth, throat, esophagus, bladder, kidney, pancreas, and lung cancer drops by up to 70 percent. Ulcers also recede

After 15 years

Many factors return to normal, as do those who have never smoked in life. In particular, conditions are equated with tooth loss, coronary heart disease, and the general risk of early death

After 20 years

The danger of getting pancreatic cancer drops to non-smoking levels. For women, the risk of death from all causes related to cigarette smoking has been shown to be as high as non-smokers

Smoke-free

After 20 years of total absence of cigarettes from your habits, you are completely free from the pathological consequences of smoking and every risk of disease is equated to that of those who have never smoked in their life.

SMOKING DISCONTINUANCE TREATMENTS

Tobacco/nicotine addiction is a chronic relapsing condition that is mostly acquired during adolescence.

Tobacco addiction has many of the characteristics of a chronic disease, so much so that most smokers persist in tobacco consumption for years or decades.

The "relapse" is considered as a return to normal tobacco consumption by a user who has stopped. Relapse typically refers to a period of several days of continuous consumption of cigarettes after a period of abstinence. Failures or relapses refer to daily tobacco consumption for at least three days after a period of at least 24 hours without smoking. A slip indicates the use of tobacco after an earlier period of abstinence, but does not result in a return to a regular habit of smoking.

This can be the case of recent ex-smokers and not who smoke less than one cigarette a day for no more than three days in a week or who smoke any number of cigarettes a day of the week, the week before a scheduled visit. A slip can be an isolated event followed by a return to abstinence, or it can be a strong predictor of relapse.

Among ex-smokers relapse is common and occurs more frequently in the first days of an attempt to quit when withdrawal symptoms are more intense. More than 75% of people who stop alone fall within the first week, making this a critical time frame to overcome.

Once patients have been smoke-free for two to three months their risk of relapse is much lower, but under no circumstances completely zeroed out. Even among tobacco users who have managed to quit for longer or shorter periods, the risk of relapse remains high. Patients who remain smoke-free for at least 12 months have a 35% chance of relapse over the course of theirlives.

Tobacco addiction may require persistent and repeated therapeutic interventions, as well as long-term follow-up to recovery.

Understanding its chronic nature implies long-term observation, and not simply the interventions that are administered during the acute stages. After the relapse, several drug treatments may be required, sometimes alternating between medications, as well as educating patients and offering them psycho-behavioral support to avoid further relapse.

No effective treatment has yet been identified to prevent relapse into tobacco addiction in the astinent smoker. Simply being an ex-smoker is not a sure guarantee of the end of tobacco addiction. Although many clinicians are able to treat patients with chronic diseases such as diabetes, high blood pressure, andtc., feel less comfortable when they have to treat tobacco addiction, because they ignore the fact that such addiction is a chronic disease.

The consideration of tobacco consumption as a chronic disease facilitates and accelerates the healing process, and increases the success rate of pharmacotherapy aimed at the cessation of nicotine dependence, and reduces relapses in tobacco consumption. We advise all healthcare professionals who assist identifiable patients such as smokers to consider tobacco consumption and addiction as a chronic relapsed disorder and to define it in medical terms as tobacco addiction.

HELP! I WANT TO SMOKE! WHAT DO I DO?

Willpower is often not enough, sometimes not even drugs are enough: sooner or later the crisis comes. What can we do to overcome it?
Let's not test ourselves
First of all let's not be "induced into temptation": let's get rid of the remaining packages, the lighters and everything that reminds us of smoking. Also clean the car, clothing and house to remove the smell of smoke that could rekindle the desire. Then make it clear to others (family, friends, colleagues) that you are trying to quit and that it would be appropriate for us not to be offered cigarettes.
Avoid the environments where you are smoking and avoid smokers (well, as far as possible... we don't want to become hermits!)

and manage situations in which smoking would be natural: after meals, in the coffee break, after an aperitif etc.
But what if the desire gets urgent? We need to find something that distracts us for about five minutes. Only five minutes: this is usually the time it takes to get through the height of the crisis. After these five very hard minutes, the desire subsides.
So what to do? How to occupy these five "cursed" minutes?
Here are some tips:
1-chew a chewing-gum or a strictly sugar-free candy.
2-drink water or a juice. Avoid sugary drinks.
3-if you really want to nibble something, address the
4-count fruit or vegetable.
5-print the reasons why it was decided to stop and reread them several times, even aloud.
6-never stand still: find something to do.

Smoking is also a ritual made of gestures: if our hands are busy (to cook, clean, work) they can not take the pack of cigarettes. Remember, it's only 5 minutes. They may look very long, but it's only 5.

How to resist the cigarette when in the company of smokers?

Avoid the company of smokers. In the early days, it is advisable to avoid the places where you smoke and to preferably frequent friends who do not smoke. Smoking-free law enforcement is a real support when you are trying to quit smoking. It is easier nowadays to attend non-smoking clubs and restaurants. Keep in mind that it is difficult to resist the urge to smoke when you smell tobacco or when you see someone lighting a cigarette.

Moderate alcohol and coffee consumption.

Many ex-smokers started smoking again after drinking alcohol, particularly in the evening. In fact, alcohol, although in limited quantities, decreases the will and increases the desire to smoke. Similarly, coffee can provoke the desire to smoke. Avoid drinking or at least be particularly careful.

Resist the influence of smokers.

Do not be influenced by people who are disturbed by your success and who want to encourage you to take your cigarette back. Tell yourself that many smokers would also like to quit. Affirm your new identity as an ex-smoker. You can respond to provocations like this, for example:

"No thanks, I got rid of this slavery."

"No thanks, I have decided not to poison myself with tobacco again."

"No thanks, I don't need cigarettes to feel good."

Repeat the scene, like an actor.

Stage in advance the moment when you refuse the cigarette that is offered to you, and the moment when you respond to a person who doubts your ability to succeed. Prepare ironic answers, this can solve a number of unpleasant situations and demolish sarcastic interventions.

THE FALLOUT: IT'S NOT A FAILURE

"Not like it happened, but I was smoking without even realizing it," "I was with friends and I couldn't resist," "Well, a cigarette you want me to do? I'm not smoking tomorrow." These other sentences are the corollary, the justification of an event: relapse (or recurrence).

The fallout should not be experienced as a defeat: on average it takes 3 to 7 attempts before you can completely stop.

It is therefore very important to avoid self-pity and discouragement, but it is necessary to analyse with clarity the causes that have led to the resumption of smoking.

For example:

When did we start again?

Was it a situation of emotional stress (grief, personal or work conflicts)?
Was it a situation of "temptation" (convivial moments, coffee break, meetings with people who smoke)?
Have I forgotten to follow the advice to overcome the crisis (e.g. drinking water, chewing gum or candy, texting or calling, eating a fruit, brushing my teeth, taking deep breaths, counting, singing, getting nails etc.)?
Have I resumed bad eating habits (e.g. coffee or alcohol use) and physical (I didn't move)?
Did I properly follow the posology of the drugs I was prescribed for smoking cessation? The analysis of the factors that induced, favored and triggered the crisis that led to the fallout will allow me, next time, to detect them in time and to avoid or minimize them. We can implement some strategies:
If you have bought cigarettes, throw them away

Avoid if possible (we are not hermits!) parties, invitations from smokers, coffee breaks with "embedded" cigarette

Practice one of the small alternative activities mentioned above in order to spend the maximum desire 5 minutes

Call your doctor

Write and read the reasons why you want to quit

Writing and reading the goals already achieved (how long we have not smoked, what has improved in our body)

Reward yourself: Set aside all or part of the money saved by giving yourself a gift. You deserved it!

The fallout is not a failure, but an opportunity to get to know each other better, fortify us and improve.

However, it is always necessary to analyse the causes of the relapse.

Relapse is a normal phenomenon, which is part of the process necessary to quit smoking. On average, ex-smokers made 4 serious attempts before they could really quit. Tell yourself that your latest attempt has allowed you to buy experience and that this will increase your chances of success next time.

What were the circumstances of my last relapse? Why did I start again?

EFFECTIVE STRATEGIES TO PREVENT RELAPSE

Do more sports or exercise

The sport frees from tensions and allows to decrease the desire to smoke. Playing sports also increases self-esteem and strengthens your new identity as a person who takes care of their health. It is a pleasant and effective way to avoid relapse.

Be active

Practice the activities you like the most. Plan your activities in advance. Be careful not to have too many dead times when cigarette regrets might creep in.

Change your environment

Avoid keeping items at your fingertips that may cause the desire to smoke. Drop the cigarette packets, hide the ashtrays and lighters. Do not carry cigarettes with you and avoid asking smokers. Wash your clothes to remove the smell of smoke.

Seeking help from people close to you

You can increase your chances of success with the support of the people around you. Let others know that you have stopped smoking and ask them to help you. Don't hesitate to talk to a trusted person about your efforts to quit smoking to a trusted person. Be wary of some smokers, they can be driven by envy for your results and encourage you to start again.

Ask for the help of a professional

The help of a professional increases your chances of success. Can:

Talk to your doctor. He will help you himself or re-orient you towards someone who can do it.

Contact an addiction specialist.

Participate in a group support program (such as a 5-day plan).

Incite your partner to quit

In two, you can share your experience and help each other. In addition, if your partner stops smoking, this increases your chances of success.

Be proud of yourself!

By quitting smoking, you have achieved a victory and regained your freedom. Be proud of your success. Be aware that it enhances you in the eyes of those who cannot stop smoking. These positive feelings can help you maintain your new position as an ex-smoker.

Giving yourself rewards

Buy gifts with the money you saved by giving up cigarettes: you really deserved them! Some rewards cost nothing, like talking to yourself in a positive way ("I'm very proud to have been able to quit smoking"), go and find friends or take time off. These rewards will encourage you to continue and reward the loss of smoking pleasure. And why not give some small gifts even to the people who are close to you, and who perhaps had to endure your irritability as an ex-smoker?

Keep two lists with you

For a few days, try to do this experiment : keep with you two lists and consult them when the urge to smoke is felt, this will replace the gesture of pulling out your pack of cigarettes :

the list of reasons why you quit smoking

the list of your personal techniques to resist the desire to smoke

Interpreting the urge to smoke as a signal

Even long after you quit smoking you should expect to feel the desire of the cigarette. Do not consider these "cravings" as failures, but as warning signs that tell you that you still have to use the strategies and techniques described in these pages.

Manage any weight gain

In general, you gain weight after quitting smoking. However, this increase is moderate (from 3 to 4 kg on average) and there are many simple and effective techniques for losing weight or avoiding buying. In particular, the use of the nicotine patch in ex-smokers allows to limit, or at least delay, weight gain. Say to yourself, "One thing at a time. For now I face my cigarette habit, then I will address the problem of weight gain. If I can quit smoking, then I will also be able to lose weight." Starting again to smoke will not necessarily make you lose weight. On the contrary, the fallout could knock you down and lead you to overeat. To limit weight gain, avoid fatty foods, exercise more and get enough sleep. Eat more fruits and vegetables. There are many books on different ways of losing weight, get advice in a good library. Ask for support from a dietician. Above all, avoid imposing too strict diets, because this would involve too many difficulties at once. Quitting smoking must be your priority. It is better to take a few kilo now than to weigh 35 in chemotherapy; If something like this happens to you, you won't even dare to hope to gain weight.

Making a list of the benefits of a tobacco-free life

Here are the benefits described as part of one of our surveys by some ex-smokers and ex-smokers.

"I spend less money."

"I feel younger." "I have more energy." "I feel fitter."

"I rediscovered the flavors and smells."

"I feel so much better." "Breathe better." "I feel a certain pride."

"I have a better breath." "The smell on the clothes is gone." "I look better."

"I don't have to worry about my lungs anymore."

"I don't cough anymore." "No more headaches." "I'm less nervous."

"The others are less disturbed." "This re-evaluates me in the eyes of the people who are close to me." "My family is satisfied."

If doubt prevails...

Prepare an answer that will allow you not to start over.

AVOID FALLING BACK IN CASE OF STRESS OR LOW MORALE

In case of low morale

Nicotine is a stimulant, so it is possible that some people feel down when they stop smoking. As well as the other symptoms of abstinence this feeling should pass after a certain period. If depression does not pass, consider this seriously and do not hesitate and consult with a doctor.

Targeting the causes of stress

Try to understand the causes of stress, then point to the root of the problem. In doing so, you will find ways to react to stress other than smoking. Regular practice of a relaxation technique (yoga, sophrology) can help you better manage stress and tension.

Relax

Slowly take several deep breaths. Relax by listening to music, talking to someone, reading a newspaper or book, doing sports, exercises or another activity you like. At least during the first few days it is advisable to sleep a lot or make some naps.

Avoid conflicts

It is recommended to avoid the causes of nervousness and conflict situations during the first weeks after quitting smoking. Always keep in mind that a cigarette never solves problems.

Engage people close to you

After quitting smoking some people become irritable. Notify the people around you and ask them to be patient and understanding for some time.

Expressing your feelings

If you talk about your emotions, they become easier to manage. Express openly and calmly what you hear. Keep in touch with your friends or loved ones by phoning and meeting them as often as possible.

Organize your time

By planning your activities in advance, you avoid moments of boredom when you can more easily insinuate the urge to smoke.

Instead of dealing with things to do in the way they come up, set priorities. Determine which hours are your most productive and dedicated to the most important tasks. Try to maintain control even if unexpected or interruptions occur (phone calls, visits, etc.) anticipating your behavior. Learn to say no. And most importantly, provide "pleasure" activities to recharge your batteries.

QUIT SMOKING: THE "SIDE EFFECTS"

Alongside the undoubted benefits of ending cigarette use, "side effects" may appear that could hamper the path to complete cigarette abandonment. On this page we will talk about the most common.

Weight gain

Is a possibility that worries everyone who wants to quit smoking. Everyone wonders "how much will I get fat?" In particular, women are asked to do so, who are more susceptible to the problem and who are often discouraged from starting or continuing a path of addiction precisely because of weight gain. But the most correct question would be, "Will I get fat?" Yes, because in reality not everyone gets fat and generally the weight gain is not

more than 2-3 kilos, if you observe some precautions.
First of all, you don't have to go on a diet! Quitting smoking involves a significant amount of willpower and there is not enough left even for a diet.
It is better to gradually change your eating habits, perhaps by looking at a few simple tips:
Eat calmly: It takes about 15 minutes to feel full, so by eating quickly we risk swallowing more food than necessary.
Increase the amount of vegetables and fruits consumed throughout the day, orient yourself towards low-caloriefoods.
When you feel the need for the cigarette, use candy or chewing-gum strictly without sugar.
Drink plenty of water, avoiding alcohol and sugarydrinks.
Increase physical activity with criterion: those who are always in the chair take a walk or a bike

ride. You don't have to run a marathon right away!

Avoid quitting smoking at Christmas, during holidays or holidays: these are occasions where you tend to eat more than you need and the lack of a cigarette could exacerbate this trend.

The constipation

Drink a lot, eat more fruits and vegetables, move more should be enough to prevent the problem. If you present yourself in a stubborn manner, you can resort to mild laxatives and possibly resort to the most energetic ones only after consulting the doctor.

Nervousness, irritability, difficulty concentrating, sleep disorders.

From half to two-thirds of people who stop smoking report one or more of these symptoms. They are due to the nicotine "abstinence crisis" but, however annoying, they are fortunately transient. However, it is advisable to avoid triggering or exacerbating them, for example

It's a chance he's going to show up... if you haven't read the previous paragraph!

Limiting the use of coffee, tea and alcohol, especially before fallingasleep.

Taking small breaks whileworking.

Drinking a herbal tea or chamomile before bed (even hot milk, but only if you digest iteasily).

Sleeping longer hours thanusual.

THE SMOKER'S DIARY

Keeping a smoker's diary helps you become aware of your addiction and correct behaviors that do not allow us to quit smoking.

There is a diary template called Five Minute Journal that was devised by Alex Ikonn and UJ Ramdas and is based on the latest research in behavioural sciences. The two have devised a diary model that can help you be more focused, have more productive days and ultimately be happier. If you don't try it for at least 5 days, it's hard to tell what I'm talking about.

There is a paper version and an application of the Five Minute Journal.

The diary is basically made up of 5 essential parts.

The first part is that of gratitude and it is filled out in the morning.

One of the most interesting things about this diary is the fact that it needs to be filled in as soon as you wake up and before bedtime. This time breakdown allows us to put the right rhythm to our days and to "program" our mind during sleep.

As for the parts to be filled out in the morning, the first is about gratitude. If we're not grateful, we can't be happy. So the first question you'll need to answer in your timeline is as follows:

What are the three things I am grateful for this morning?

No deep or mystical answers, you just have to write three little things for which you are grateful.

The second part of the diary, always to be filled in in the morning, is about your priorities for the day.

Specifically, you need to answer this simple question:

What are the three activities that will make today a great day?
Project your mind in the evening and imagine that you have completed these three activities, activities that make you feel good, activities that help you grow. Would it be a well-spent day or not?

Writing these 3 most important activities in the morning also has the power to influence that portion of our brains that are responsible for filtering information from the outside environment. Put simply, focusing on the 3 activities you just wake up to, it will help you be active for the rest of the day.

After writing priorities for your day, in the third part of the diary (always to be filled in in the morning), we will report the medium-term goals (3-5 years).

The question you need to answer is the following:

Who will I have become from here to 5 years old?

The goal of this third part is to help you visualize your goals. For visualization to have a real effect, however, you don't just have to write down your future life, you also need to briefly imagine the process that will have allowed you to achieve these goals.

You don't have to come up with new goals every morning. Once you have written them on the first day, repeat the exact same phrases every blessed morning. These goals must become almost a mantra.

Once you've completed the first 3 parts of your diary, set it aside and start your day. Then resume it in the evening, before going to sleep. In fact, there are 2 other short parts to complete, but extremely important.

The fourth section of this effective diary template covers those events of the day that made you happy. Our happiness, in fact, depends not only on what happens to us, but also on our ability to become aware of it.

In the evening, answer this first question:

What were three wonderful things that happened today?

I know, there are shitty days when everything seems to go wrong. Yet even in these days, if we strive a little bit, we will always find some beautiful: a smile, a flavor, a scent, a moment.

The fifth part of our diary is really interesting and it's about what we can still improve. To close your journal, you'll need to answer this last question:

How could I have made today a better day?

Orienting our mind towards improvement, just before bedtime, is an exceptionally powerful tool to ensure that our subconscious reworks at night the best strategies to improve our lives, day after day (or rather: night after night).

STRATEGIES TO AVOID WEIGHT GAIN

The lack of nicotine causes urgent desires to smoke that tend to subside with food. The solution is to avoid sedentary, walk, run, move, dance. Do the things you like to "forget" the need to compensate with smoking: love, reading, gardening and any other pleasant activity. Help yourself with nicotinic substitutes that calm the craving and allow you to better understand your food mechanisms by correcting them. It is useless to start a diet, because this would only add stress to the stress. However, it is useful to review the basic principles of good nutrition.

Eat in various ways: expand the choice of your food. A balanced diet is a varied diet, rich in nutritional elements but low in calories.

Take many cereals and potatoes : wholemeal bread, pasta, cereals and potatoes are practically fat-free, but they have many vitamins, minerals, oligo-elements and fiber. Accompany them with other foods that are low in fat.

Prefer fruits and vegetables – 5 portions a day of fruit and/or vegetables, fresh, steamed or in the form of juice (1 serving, a full handful, a glass of juice).

Eat milk or dairy products and fish once or twice a week; consumption of meat and eggs is moderate; these foods contain important nutritional elements such as calcium in milk, iodine, selenium, omega 3 fatty acids in freshwater fish. Meat contains iron, vitamins B1, B6 and B12. Between 300 and 600 g. of meat per week are sufficient. Preferably consume meat and dairy products with a few fatty materials.

Take low fat : use rather vegetable oils and fats (e.g. rapeseed oil or soybeans). Pay attention to fats in meat, dairy products, butter, pastry products, confectionery and finished products and avoid fast-food. Our body does not need more than 70-90 gr. fat per day.

Consume moderately sugar and salt: do not consume any sugary foods or beverages (e.g. glucose syrup). As an alternative to salt, use spices creatively in the kitchen. Or else you prefer iodized salt. Drink a lot of water : water is vital. Drink 1.5 litres a day.

Choose natural water. Do not consume alcoholic beverages except in moderation and occasionally.

Prepare your meals carefully: cook at a low temperature, without letting things cook for a long time and with little water and fat. In this way you will preserve the natural taste of the foods and the nutritional elements that are contained in it.

Take the time to enjoy your dish : have the thigh of what you eat. Eat with your eyes, and slowly. You will gain in pleasure, your senses will be more alive and you will soon feel full.

Do not snack : it is advisable to limit yourself to three meals a day, according to the principle "to have breakfast as an emperor- to have lunch like a king- and to dine like a beggar". It is preferable that breakfast and lunch are high in fiber and that dinner, rich rather in protein, is eaten early in the evening.

Weight Gain Considerations

Former smokers become more numerous every day; they're the obese.

Weight gain is a very frequent concern for those who decide to quit tobacco smoking. It is common to gain weight after quitting smoking and although it is kilos that can be removed with some effort, in the immediate are difficult to accept. Therefore, many smokers wonder if it is worth the effort to quit smoking if, then, to reduce the risks related to smoking you increase those related to being overweight. The answer comes from a study published in the Journal of the American Medical Association and is clear: Quitting smoking always pays off. Research that followed more than 3,000 volunteers for 25 years showed that despite weight gain following smoking cessation, people who abandoned tobacco had a lower risk of incurring a lower cardiovascular event than more than 50% of those who continued to smoke. So the advice is to accept a few extra pounds, knowing that then the excess weight accumulated will go away soon.

So, if you are following a path to quit smoking it is important to observe food rules and frequently it is necessary to change some habits also in view of the fact that the type of diet that makes the smoker can often make more difficult to stop smoking.

Smoking and eating usually represent for the smoker the types of gratification easier approach: so it is normal that if smoking is lost he tends to move more on food.

It's only fair to reward yourself with something as rewarding as food, but to do so so that it's more beneficial in terms of health and cessation of smoking you need to pay attention to some general tips:

-privilege some foods (generally low-calorie and fighting the pleasure of smoking) rather than others (especially avoiding the so-called "junk food")

-engage in food preparation and don't just think about consuming it

-Make the dishes attractive to the eye; presentation adds value to what we've prepared

-it is good to give us what we like and even with a certain frequency, as long as it is small quantities; feeding the sense of deprivation can lead us sooner or later to binge

-if our favorite food gratification is sweets avoid eating them fasting, but at the end of the meal.

In addition, to effectively counteract any weight gain that often occurs after quitting smoking, physical activity can be increased.

I note that activating the gratification circuit through food is one of the mechanisms on which the smoker more easily tends to fall back once the nicotinic stimulus is lost, it is inevitable that if gratification is shifted reckless and impulsive on food, you risk taking extra pounds.
Let's take an example to better understand how repeated but small rewards in terms of palate pleasures, can help us change our daily rhythms that have been punctuated by cigarettes for years.

If we want to train a dog to come to us every time we say its name, it must be associated with the behavior (rush) associated with a gratification (a bite of meat). So we can train him by rushing it once a day and rewarding it with a big steak, or we can cut the steak into small bites and repeat the process several times throughout the day. With the second method, the dog will learn much faster and better the action of flocking when called.

Equally, if we want to learn to exclude smoking from our daily habits, we must balance cigarette renunciation behaviour with other activities that give us gratification. And the most effective way to do this is to barter the renunciation of smoking with small and repeated pleasures (e.g. sugar-free gums and candies, liquorice sticks, etc.).

The pleasure brain circuit is a memory circuit and therefore if we activate it constantly and in a controlled way it will be easier to comply with the new provisions that stipulate to exclude smoking from our daily habits.

We certainly can't replace every unsomoled cigarette with pastries and chocolates.

Proper lifestyles and healthy eating are important prevention measures because they produce far greater benefits than the use of drugs or other medical-surgical equipment.

Assisted smoking cessation interventions should also address the issues of healthy and more appropriate eating to counterbalance metabolic re-adjustment resulting from the elimination of smoking especially if there is a pre-existing problem of excess weight. It is therefore important to prevent the beneficial effects of the abolition of smoking from being reversed by the negative effects of obesity, which, like smoking, also robs the individual on average of 9 years of life. So, after you have passed the critical stages of smoking cessation and you are in a situation of prolonged complete remission, it is important to comply with the rule of not associating food with rewards or punishments, but food should be limited to just enough to stay healthy.

Smoking cessation, provided it is dealt with seriously, is generally associated with a subsequent phase of food change that prioritises the consumption of fruits and vegetables and a phase of lifestyle change towards greater physical activity. Moreover, fruits and vegetables have a protective action especially against lung and mouth cancers that represent structures of the body often attacked by tobacco smoke. On the basis of this information, it is useful to accompany the cessation of smoking to a concomitant intervention on the diet provided that it is well accepted by the person concerned and is not perceived as restrictive or limiting, but rather as a stimulant and Enriching. It is therefore important to focus on the feeding factor, which is certainly a valuable aid in the fight against smoking.

THE 10 LEGENDS THE SMOKER CAN'T GET RID OF

People start smoking for many reasons. Many continue to snort because they believe (or want to believe) in certain legends about tobacco use. Here are 10 of these myths, and the truth about each of them.

Myth 1: My other healthy habits can do for my smoking.

Some smokers justify their habit by insisting that proper nutrition and exercise are enough to keep them healthy. It's not like that. "Research shows that a healthy diet and exercise do not reduce the health risks associated with smoking," says Ann M. Malarcher, PhD, scientific consultant at the CDC's Office on Smoking and Health. 'Smoking affects every system in the body, and to think that finding the perfect lifestyle to counteract the effects of smoking is unrealistic.'

Myth 2: Switching to "light" cigarettes will reduce my risk.

Smokers who switch to "light" and "mild" cigarettes will inevitably compensate for low levels of tar and nicotine by inhaling smoke more deeply or smoking more.

Myth 3: I've been smoking for a long time; the damage is already done.

The damage caused by smoking is cumulative, and the longer a person smokes, the greater the risk of contracting life-threatening diseases. But quitting smoking at any age brings health benefits. "Your health will improve, even if you stop at 70," says Norman H. Edelman, MD, chief medical officer of the American Lung Association. The benefits of quitting start as early as the day you stop. Within a year, the risk of having a heart attack will be reduced by 50%. According to the American Cancer Society, smokers who quit before the age of 35 at the risk of smoking-related health problems. A smoker who quits before the age of 50 halves the risk of dying within the next 15 years compared to those who continue to smoke.

Myth 4: Trying to quit smoking stresses me out and this is not healthy.

True, quitting smoking is stressful, but there is no evidence that a period of stress has long-term negative effects. In fact, research shows that smokers who quit start eating better, exercising more and feeling better about themselves. Today, many smokers today hate the fact that they are addicted to cigarettes and also that they are taking money away from the family budget to throw them "in smoke".

Myth 5: The weight gain that hurts when you stop smoking is just as bad as smoking.

Smokers who stop "earning" on average 5-6 kg. But the health risk due to the extra pounds is lower than the risk of continuing to smoke, in addition the weight gain is transient and can be contained with proper nutrition and proper exercise (among other things, easier precisely thanks to abandonment of cigarettes).

Myth 6: The only way to stop is to do it all of a sudden thanks to willpower.

Some smokers think that "cold turkey" is the best approach and that willpower is the only effective tool to curb tobacco cravings. This is only partially true: willpower and commitment are essential, but smokers are more likely to be able to quit if they take advantage of counselling services and medications for the treatment of smoking drugs, including nicotine (gums, patches, pads, inhaler, or nasal spray) and prescription drugs: bupropion, varenicline and cytisine). "Counseling" increases the chances of success by 60%, and taking medication doubles the odds.

Myth 7: Nicotine products are as harmful as smoking.

Nicotine is safe when used directly as a drug. Even using nicotine every day for years would be less harmful than smoking. Cigarettes provide nicotine along with 4,000 other compounds, including more than 60 known carcinogens

Myth 8: Smoking cuts is pretty good.

Reducing the number of cigarettes is not an effective strategy: smokers who reduce cigarettes suck more deeply and smoke every cigarette to the end. So even if they smoke fewer cigarettes, they take the same dose of toxic smoke. The data suggest that the only effective strategy for quitting smoking is "not even a shot."

Myth 9: I am the only one harmed by my smoking.

Tobacco smoke also harms people around you. In the United States, the American Lung Association estimates that passive smoking causes about 50,000 deaths a year. It has been estimated that a waiter who works an eight-hour shift in a smoky bar aspires as much toxic smoke as a packet smoker a day.

Myth 10: I tried to quit once and I failed, so it's useless to try again.

Most smokers try several times before always quitting. So if you've failed before, don't be put off by trying again. Whenever the person tries to quit, he learns things that might be useful for the next attempt. We like to say that the first or second time you try it is a workout and that the third or fourth time you can do it well. We need to keep trying.

SMOKING THE FIRST CIGARETTE

What does it take to become a regular smoker? Often a cigarette is enough. Recent research has analysed numerous surveys identifying the eight that most closely matched the selection criteria and which most represented the adult population.
Overall, 216314 respondents were considered, of whom 60.3% smoked at least once.
In this portion of respondents, as many as 68.9% had subsequently switched, at least temporarily, to daily smoking.
The most significant aspect of this result concerns the implications in the youth population: with a "conversion rate" potentially equal to two-thirds of tobacco users, a strong disincentive policy and a strong disincentive policy and a strong disincentive

policy is evident and necessary. increased efforts for even the occasional smoking among teens.

FALSE CIGARETTE MYTHS

Smoking a "like" cigarette.

In the face of the undoubted benefits of cigarette abandonment, the smoker likes his cigarette, enjoys the aroma, flavor, sensory differences between the brands, its being the ideal conclusion of a meal or a coffee break. And around this "pleasure" he has built, perhaps helped by a more or less obvious corporate marketing, a series of false myths, beautiful images and some authentic... dance!

Let's look at some of them:

Do you want to put the charm of the "beautiful dark" or the "femme fatale" with a cigarette between your fingers?

Yellowish fingers, ruined teeth, heavy breath, grayish and wrinkled skin, reddened eyes, smelly hair... are these the characteristics of fascinating people?

I'm becoming an adult: smoking is "grown up", from "mature" people
A classic! But, look at it, you start smoking because "everyone does it." And many greetings to maturity...
Smoking relaxes me.
Since nicotine deficiency in smoker causes withdrawal symptoms, including nervousness and irritability, it is obvious that taking additional nicotine with the cigarette calms these sensations.
It is a dog bites its tail: I take a substance whose lack causes me nervousness that pushes me to take that substance again. In short: addiction.
Smoking improves sex
Research shows that the risk of impotence increases in smoking males. Nicotine-related vasocostrition and poor oxygenation due to carbanio monoxide reduce the ability to achieve and maintain an erection. In women,

the genitals are less sprayed and therefore less sensitive. Smoking also reduces fertility rates.

Cancer? Infarction? But if my grandfather (or uncle, cousin, friend etc.) smoked 2 packets a day and went up to 95 years old! Like a swallow doesn't make spring, a grandfather... it doesn't do statistics! It is anti-scientific (or simply foolish) to base a judgment on a single or a few cases. Smoking does not give the certainty of developing cancer or having a heart attack, but it is a certainty that smokers have a significantly higher incidence of oncological and cardiovascular diseases than non-smokers.

So: you can get to old age even by smoking, but you have to see in what conditions you get there!

Stop? At my age? The damage has now been done...

Quitting smoking brings short- and long-term

benefits (links), some subjectively and easily perceived.

FIND THE REASON TO STOP FROM THE STORIES

Inserting a series of smoking cessation stories serves each of the readers in order to seek a motivation to do the same thing. Telling and listening are two very important verbs in life. Sometimes having the availability to listen means that you are willing to let your life change. Knowing how to tell something important and knowing how to listen to those who tell: in this mutual listening, each becomes bread for the other, we become support for one another, thus changing our relationships and also our lives. The act of learning is the act of acquiring knowledge and it is on the basis of knowledge that we can learn, act and strive to improve.

1° Story

"Hi everyone, I am 33 years old, and I completely stopped smoking at the age of 30. I state that I have been smoking since I was 20 years old and that I have been smoking 20 cigarettes daily for the past five years. I was certainly not an occasional or moderate smoker, the nicotine, the ritual of the cigarette at any time and in any place, were events that deeply marked my day. In September 2018, I came across an offer of a well-known Italian airline, which allowed you to go to the beach in Kenya with 700 euros all-inclusive. I thought there were so many to spend, but I calculated that I was paying, or rather I threw the same amount in just 7/8 weeks of smoking! The cigarette, hoping that the excuse should not be a bad disease. Between myself and me, I made the following reasoning: I spend these 500 euros and quit smoking to recover them in less than two meters and yes. But how will I do it?

Simple: the day I leave for Kenya, I get up in the morning, I avoid smoking with a bit of willpower, I run to the airport (and it will be more than 12 hours that I will not have burned), I embark and, from that moment, I already know that I will not be able to burn for about 12 hours (9-10 hours of travel in addition to the time required to complete all customs formalities, collect baggage, exit the airport and reach the city and the hotel). Then there will be tiredness, the time zone, the excitement of having landed in another world, all factors that distract you much, and almost make you not think of cigarettes. You won't believe it, but in this way, I arrived at 48 hours of abstinence without realizing it. The fact of having moments of crisis was attenuated in my head by the point of not being able to have cigarettes, or not being able to buy them, or not being able to smoke them in the place where I was at that moment. In the following days, I was able to maintain without problems faith in my goal because, in the place where I found the cigarettes, it was hard enough. Since I had taken the road to cessation, I didn't even bother to understand how I could do to get them. The moments of abstinence with the passing of the days became less present. I spent a week without smoking, and at the end of the week, I also felt better physically. It may have been the sea air or something else, or only the pack of cigarettes, but my physique seemed different. I can assure you that for me, it was all about the head. If you are convinced and determined to want to quit, choose the right period or the one in which you will have the opportunity to carry out an activity that gives you pleasure. You move away from work stress or everyday life (in my case, it was the trip), and you will see that after the first 2-3 days in which you will have some slight decompensation due to physical dependence, it will be much easier for you to quit. In my opinion, it would also be essential to start or intensify a physical activity appropriate to individual and personal physical conditions and possibilities. As I have read, movement and sport activity, in addition to distracting the mind, favor the production of substances that give the perception of well-being. Another thing that helped me over a long period from the day the smoke was quit was a simple application on the phone. Through this application, I can still see the state of improvement of my physique, the number of cigarettes not smoked, the money saved by not smoking, and other exciting information. I assure you that after a few years, the numbers become impressive, and you notice how much you can smoke in a lifetime. I don't know if you've ever tried to think about how many cigarettes you've smoked over the years. Do the math; perhaps this will be the spring that will help you stop. "

2° Story

"Hi everyone, I have quit smoking for seven months. I have smoked 25 cigarettes a day for almost 15 years, half of them I have spent smoking promising myself that I will have to quit as soon as possible, not to find myself maybe one day in having to do it after a diagnosis of cancer or some other smoking-related disease. I smoked without satisfaction in the past ten years; I honestly thought that cigarettes did not taste good. I smoked convinced that this vice would bring me to the grave, that I would never have been able to give up cigarettes, always putting them first of all, sometimes before even my wife. I felt like a cigarette slave, and more and more, I tried to find the system to replace it with something to be able to get rid of it without too much suffering, the years went by, and the feeling of not being able to get rid of them increased. The fear of irreparably compromising my health over the years has increased, slow nte ed inexorably. I've always wondered in various attempts where the mistake was. I was probably wrong in looking for something to replace it at all costs because I was convinced that it should be so. Initially, I thought that the cigarette served to calm me down, but in reality, over the years, I realized that it was not so. Indeed it was just the opposite; the cigarette brought me a lot of extra anxiety. The reality is that the cigarette is a hellish trap, it makes us believe that smoking relaxes and is a pleasure, when instead it is precisely she who gives us a state of anxiety as soon as the level of nicotine in our body drops. So to restore the nicotine level, we go back to smoking. The other big mistake I made was never set a date for the last cigarette. Still, I kept alternating periods when one morning I got up saying today I don't smoke, and regularly either postponed to another day later in time or I was looking for to hold back and smoke as little as possible for then find myself after three days to recover by working overtime. You are wondering how did I quit! If I look back, I can say that it was not so difficult. The first step was to understand that I needed help to be able to quit because mine was a real addiction. I decided to rely on a doctor, who prescribed me acupuncture sessions to decrease the urge to smoke, combined with a drug treatment of a few weeks, which replaced the nicotine to be able to stop the states of withdrawal. The second point was to inform my family of my decision to quit on that particular day. Everyone helped to help me. I must say that after a few days, the states of crisis had significantly diminished. Now I have to be very careful not to let my guard down. Very often I would like to smoke one. I try to convince myself that so much one cannot do anything to me, and instead, I know very well that that cigarette could bring me back to the state of a few months ago, and when I return to reasoning, I understand that I must not do it. Here is my real problem are precisely these small drops in concentration, which I have been able to combat right now. At the moment, I can have considerable help also from my family who wants me to stop smoking again, both my wife and my children have been wonderful. I'm slowly learning to hate the cigarette; I'm trying to learn and memorize all the negative sides to repeat them in these moments of small crisis. I made a culture about the harm that smoke brings. I also think that I got rid of the stench that cigarettes bring on you, and the fetid breath they create for you. Now when I have a business meeting with other smokers, I realize how bad their breath is. Throw away all the cigarettes that you have around the house and in the car, in the garage, cellar, workplace. Don't try to make tough men who quit with cigarettes in your pocket or drawer because you will fail. To succeed, you must eliminate any temptation. For the youngest and also the youngest, keep in mind that the smartest is the one who does not smoke, and the most idiotic is the one who smokes! Good luck to all."

3°Story

"I am a 58-year-old carpenter. On my birthday I decided to quit, I was 52 years old. I started smoking before I was 14 years old. On the advice of my wife, who is a nurse at a private clinic, I went to a psychotherapist, which, with a session of just 30 minutes, helped me to achieve the goal I had set myself. Through a series of hypnosis sessions, I faced the physical discomfort due to the lack of nicotine. In the first few weeks, the pain was gone, and only I occasionally had slight anxiety attacks. After the first month, I must say that I gained a few pounds in weight. I started doing sports so as not to increase excessively. At the beginning, I took a few walks daily; then after some time, I started with a few small runs, today I run daily for about 7-8 km. I have never been a great sportsman, but I must say that such a distance after a few months of progressive training is not co, yes challenging to reach. The important thing is that since I started doing sports, the moments of crisis have almost completely gone. I recommend everyone to stop as soon as possible, and at any age, you are in your life, because smoking doesn't make any sense. "

4° Story

"I have quit smoking for a couple of years. I am a 43-year-old housewife. I smoked about 25 cigarettes a day. All I was doing was smoking. I was smoking because I was bored at home all day. Initially, I did the housework and went to the garden to smoke; then, over time, I went to smoke directly in the house until I put the beds and kitchen. In the evening, my husband got furious about the stench that remained in the house. Sometimes I used to pretend that I was smoking outside, but now I was used to smoking some of them even in the house. One evening in January, my husband arrived home and, as usual, got angry because the stench was great. That day I smoked a few more at home because it was cold outside. This time, however, my husband was so angry that he packed his bag and left the house for a week. I didn't see him for a week. I decided it was time to quit. I took a medical course (with cytisine drug) for about a month, I also did some acupuncture session, and today I am part of a group of ex-smokers who meet weekly. I recovered the relationship with my husband; everything came back as at the beginning of our story. Fantastic to have stopped! "

OTHER METHODOLOGIES: ACUPUNCTURE AND LASER

There are some practices that can help in the path of quit tuxedo with cytisine.

The acupuncture technique used to quit smoking is considered an effective remedy and absolutely free of side effects if you want to try this way in the hope of being able to quit smoking. It is a holistic practice that is part of the Chinese medical discipline, in which precise points of the body are stimulated by the surface insertion of thread-like and disposable needles in such a way as to stimulate your energy channels by strengthening your will and reducing the appetite for nicotine by restoring the balance of well-being. In practice, your body's energies are balanced in order to eliminate the need for nicotine. The practice of acupuncture to quit smoking more widespread is called Acudetox and is based on stimulation of certain parts of the ear.

Of course it is not a magic or a witchcraft, and the needle is not a magic wand. However, it's definitely a way of making your choice to quit smoking a possible perspective. The therapy must of course be accompanied by personal motivation, in fact the answer to this practice is always subjective, however it is proven that it helps to quell the hyperexcited nervous system in abstinence syndrome. Indeed, some people ensure that acupuncture has changed the taste of smoking to make it suddenly extremely unpleasant. If you want to quit smoking with all your heart, you could give her a chance!

Researchers from the Cochrane Collaboration analysed 22 published studies around the world on the use of acupuncture to quit smoking.

Different techniques

Faced with the wide variety of treatment techniques, the researchers decided to include in the study experiments on the use of needles, electrified or not, of low-dose laser beams, and of hand pressures (in this case rather than acupuncture). Some of these treatments have been carried out as part of medical consultations; the others were made by placing a device on the ear of the person intending to quit smoking. This dipositive penetrated the ear through a needle or exerted a simple pressure by means of a grain. In both cases, patients had to operate or manipulate the device from the moment they perceived the symptoms of abstinence.

Selection criteria for the study

In order to be considered by the Cochrane team, the studies had to involve a witness group, i.e. people who were not given any treatment, or a different treatment, or even a 'placebo' treatment. In the latter case, it was a question of applying needles or carrying out hand pressure in parts of the body other than those believed to be involved in tobacco addiction. In the case of laser therapy, the witness group was treated with an off device. Another condition for the study to be considered valid: that the smoking or non-smoking status was established 6 to 12 months after surgery, and that this statute was confirmed biochemically (cotinine test or exhaled carbon monoxide test) . In all cases patients had to receive treatment, or on the contrary be attributed to the witness group, at random (by draw by lot).

Results

Laser or electrostimulation treatments showed no effectiveness. At first, "classic" acupuncture proves more effective than the total absence of treatment. But the effect does not last : six months after the start of treatment, most of the people treated had fallen back into smoking and the gap with people who had not actually received the treatment (witness group) disappeared. It is therefore possible that acupuncture helps to withstand withdrawal symptoms, but one of the studies analysed showed that the effect was identical even if the stings were carried out in parts of the body other than those believed to have a specific role compared to this process. In summary, it was not possible to demonstrate a positive effect of acupuncture on tobacco disomancy processes. In essence these techniques help and integrate the process with cytisine but you still need the medical pathway with cytisine to arrive at a fairly certain result. Although there is certainly nothing if you do not have great fortitude.

THE SECOND CHOICE: REDUCING SMOKING

Smoking reduction is proposed as a second-choice option for smokers who are not willing to quit completely or who are unable to do so. The reduction in smoking should be seen as an intermediate step towards a subsequent cessation of those smokers who are unable or who do not want to quit smoking. The goal for all tobacco users remains the complete cessation of smoking. The benefits of the reduction in the approach to smoking are twofold: with the reduction of smoking, at least some of the risks decrease. It increases the patient's confidence in his ability to quit completely and increases the number of attempts in a year. The reduction in smoking has raised concerns that the smoking rate could decrease the smoking rate. There is no data to support this hypothesis; the opposite effect has even been observed. A review by the Chocrane Collaboration found no difference in the likelihood of termination between abruptly quitting and quitting having first reduced cigarette consumption, and concluded that it may be left to patients to choose to quit stop with both methods. It was observed that patients who did not want to quit were more likely to do so after a year, if they were only offered to reduce consumption and not to quit abruptly. It has been established that "smoking reduction" means a 50% decrease in initial cigarette consumption, but without complete abstinence.

A limited number of data (from small studies, selected populations and for short follow-up periods) suggest that a substantial reduction in smoking would decrease many cardiovascular risk factors and improve respiratory symptoms. Smoking reduction is associated with a 25%

decrease in tobacco bio-markers and the incidence of lung cancer and a low, almost insignificant, increase in birth weight, of babies born to smoking mothers. If smoking is reduced, there do not appear to be significant improvements in lung function. Smoking reduction is a therapeutic alternative for smokers who are not yet ready to quit completely. In a study analysing the use of nicotine gum and which observed double and triple cessation rates at 3 and 12 months respectively towards placebo, the concomitant reduction in cigarette consumption was well tolerated and led to significant reduction of the carbon monoxide biomarker. The randomised ROSCAP-controlled study, which involved reducing smoking in heart patients, assessed the effectiveness of the smoking reduction strategy in reducing harmful effects due to tobacco exposure.

The results of the study showed how those men who consumed more than the control group were able to reduce tobacco consumption. Reducing smoking with nicotine replacement The reduction of smoking with nicotine replacement therapy is recommended only in a smoker with physical dependence, i.e. a smoker in which the large number of nicotinic receptors and their desensitization is a significant factor compared to consumption, among those smokers with a Fagerstrom test score of more than 3 or even greater than 6. The reduction in smoking should be systematically proposed to highly dependent smokers, with a score of 7 or more in the Fagerstrom test, who have a tobacco-related disease and who are not ready to quit smoking. A meta-analysis of seven randomized and controlled trials involving 2767 smokers, initially not motivated to quit, showed that the withdrawal rate six months after the onset of treatment was significantly higher in smokers at NRT replacement therapy (nicotine gum, inhaler or patch) was randomly assigned for six months or more while attempting to reduce the number of cigarettes, compared to smokers in the control group: 9% vs 5%. Nicotine replacement therapy is used to replace the number of daily cigarettes reduced and therefore the harmful effects of tobacco products (other than nicotine) are potentially reduced. The more nicotine is administered more progressively, the less addiction is maintained. Pharmacological nicotine will gradually increase to a reduction of at least 50% in the number of cigarettes smoked and can be increased to get to stop.

THE DAMAGE CAUSED BY SMOKING

Gender-specific consequential damage:

Lung cancerA equal amount of tobacco consumed, the risk of lung cancer for women increases by 28 times, for men increases "only" by about 10 times; Lung cancer also occurs on average five years earlier in women. In men the frequency of lung cancer decreases, while in women it shows a steady increase.

Sexuality and fertility Smoking affects sexuality and fertility in both women and men. For this reason the cigarette is also called "hidden contraception". In women who smoke, menopause comes about 2 years earlier. Smokers taking oral contraceptives have a much higher risk of contracting cardiovascular disease, as well as an increased risk of infertility. In men smoking leads most often to erectile dysfunction and decreases the quantity and quality of sperm.

Eyes and vision disorders

Smoking is the main risk factor for retinal degeneration in relation to age. As we age, light-sensitive visual cells atrophy. The result is a disturbance in reading, difficulty in adapting light-darkness, etc. Smoking greatly promotes these irreversible aging processes.

Skin and wound healing

Smoking is the main risk factor for retinal degeneration in relation to age. As we age, light-sensitive visual cells atrophy. The result is a disturbance in reading, difficulty in adapting light-darkness, etc. Smoking greatly promotes these irreversible aging processes.20 cigarettes per day smoked in middle age lead to an early aging process of about 10 years. Tobacco smoking accelerates the normal skin aging process in several directions: it hinders collagen synthesis and thickening of individual fibers.

The reduced level of vitamin A, caused by smoking and free radicals of tobacco smoke, also activate the enzyme activity of the metalprotein-1 (MMP-1), which leads to collagen degeneration. At the same time, due to enhanced activity of the enzyme elastasis, smoking stimulates excessive degeneration of the elastin in the dermis. The vasocostrict effect of nicotine also increases tissue ischemia and accelerates skin aging.

Smoking affects the healing of wounds and fractures: in fact, the vasocostrict effect of nicotine causes a reduced proliferation of the red blood cells necessary for healing and the defense of infections, since it alters the ability of fibroblasts and macrophages of immunocompetent tissues. Nicotine also increases the aggregation of thrombocytes, which again affects microcirculation. Carbon monoxide leads to cellular hypoxia or anoxia.

The reduced new formation of collagen slows wound healing.

Finally, smoking increases the risk of various skin diseases, especially if the immunological consequences of smoking come into play. Therefore smoking triggers an inflammatory reaction in the presence of palm-plantar pustolosis, psoriasis, acne vulgaris and reverse, atopic dermatitis and obliterant thromboangitis. In the case of a malignant transformation of a human papilloma virus (HPV) infection, substances contained in tobacco are considered co-cancerous agents. In smokers, acne is significantly higher (41%) non-smokers (25%) and its resistance increases in relation to the amount of nicotine taken.

Fertility of man

Cigarette smoking is a very important risk factor in the development of both atherosclerosis and erectile dysfunction of the penis. A major Massachusetts Male Aging

Study (MMAS) found that cigarette smoking greatly amplifies the risk of impotence, especially when associated with cardiovascular disease and related drug therapies. In those aged 40 to 70, the incidence of impotence ranged from 5% to 15%. In patients treated for a heart condition, the probability of complete impotence was 56% among smokers and 21% among non-smokers. Among hypertensive patients in medical therapy, those who smoked had a full rate of impotence of 20%, while non-smokers had an 8.5% risk of impotence, comparable to that of the general population (9.6%).

Of course, not all smokers are powerless, although tobacco is harmful both for the erection and for the quality of the seminal fluid. But tobacco does not only have a harmful effect at the vascular level, favoring the formation of atheisms in all arteries, it also has a direct role on the erectile tissue of the penis.

The elasticity of the erectile tissue and therefore its ability to dilate decreases in heavy smokers, who often have a much less durable erection. This negative effect has been verified in numerous experimental studies that have shown that smoking a single cigarette can damage the quality of an erection. Elimination of cigarette smoking (present in 75% of those who came to our observation for Erectile Dysfunction) in this pathology should therefore be considered the first-line therapy of erectile dysfunction, as well as one of the most important measures in the prevention of atherosclerosis. For the doctor, moreover, the therapy of erectile dysfunction of the penis is the most important argument to induce a patient to quit smoking. The prospect of improving sexual performance is a very strong motivation to make the smoker abandon his drug addiction. Smoking can also reduce fertility by reducing sperm density, sperm count and mobility.

Fertility of the woman

Smokers have a much more frequent incidence of infertility due to hormonal causes because smoking reduces the woman's natural fertility. Smokers are exposed to an increased risk of tubaric pregnancies and pregnant women at an increased risk of miscarriages, premature births, early rupture of fetal membranes, placenta previa and premature detachment of the placenta.

Osteoporosis

Tobacco consumption leads to a reduction in bone density due to changes in the hormonal and cellular levels. It affects bone structure in menopausal women, regardless of the hormonal situation. Nicotine decreases the concentration in the serum of vitamin D and paratormone, thus affecting the balance of calcium. Particularly in individuals from the age of 50, smoking is accompanied by a significant reduction in bone mass and a consequent increased risk of fracture.

SIDS (SUDDEN INFANT DEATH SYNDROME) or sudden infant death

The sudden death of the infant, with a percentage of 25%, represents in industrialized countries the leading cause of death in the age of 1 to 12 months in the postneonatal period. A systematic review of 29 case-control studies and ten cohorts showed a doubling of the risk of SIDS due to smoking in pregnancy in 1997. Smoking of parents after birth also increases the risk of SIDS.

Vitamin C deficiency

Vitamin C assimilation in the smoker is about 10% lower, and the need for antioxidants increases by about 40%. Therefore smokers have an increased vitamin C requirement of 50% (150 mg/d).

Tooth support apparatus (parade)

Multiple cross-cutting studies, as well as long-term prospective studies, have also confirmed cigarette smoking as an important risk factor for the onset and progression of damage to paradontal tissue. Smoking is a significant risk factor for diseases of the tooth support apparatus, it also leads to the fall of teeth and causes cancer in the oral cavity and guinea pig. Smoking worsens vascularization of the oral cavity. Particularly insidious is that smoking inhibits bleeding gums, which is a typical signal of paradontitis and a wake-up call for the disease. More than 70% of dental patients with chronic paradontic disease are smokers. Compared to non-smokers, they have a risk of about 5-6 times greater; Heavy smokers, who have been smoking more than 20 cigarettes a day for more than 20 years, are at up to 20 times as high a risk of the disease. Smokers have significantly more sick and deep gum pockets, a greater loss of bone tissue and connectiveness surrounding the tooth and are more exposed to tooth loss. Compared to non-smokers, the success of treatment of dental paradontitis therapy among smokers is much more negative, as a result most failures are recorded among those in this category.

Relationship between smoking and dementia

Recent studies show that smoking, over time, increases the risk of mental problems. According to a group of researchers at the University of London, smoking vice, if prolonged for a long time (even during the so-called "silver age"), greatly increases the risk of mental decline. The results of the research showed that smokers are more prone to damage to blood vessels, including brain vessels. Smoking, once introduced, causes a narrowing and hardening of the arteries, compromising the supply of oxygen to the brain. The "cigarette vice", therefore, with the passing of the years, does not only damage bronchi and lungs; on the contrary, it also seems to affect and deteriorate brain functions.

Stroke

It manifests itself with loss of consciousness, loss of feces and urine. It can lead to death or result in paralysis of a part of the body. Stroke is the third leading cause of death in the U.S. and is also very common in Italy. The risk of accidents of this kind increases by twice or four times among smokers. By quitting smoking, the risk is reduced drastically after a year. After 5-10 years it becomes superimposed on that of those who have never smoked.

EFFECTS OF PASSIVE SMOKING ON HEALTH

Numerous rigorous studies have shown that air pollution is responsible for 1/4 of respiratory diseases. Exposure to environmental tobacco smoke (FTA) is now widely demonstrated, according to the Enviromental Protectonio Agency (EPA) "one of the most widespread and dangerous air pollutants in neighbouring environments"(3) a significant health risk for non-smokers. The Surgeon General of the USA and the National Academy of Sciences concluded that passive smoking is also able to induce lung cancer in smokers and that the children of smoking parents have a higher incidence of pneumonia, bronchitis and asthmatic seizures than children of non-smoking parents. According to these reports, passive smoking causes almost 5,000 lung cancer deaths in non-smokers each year in the US. In Italy, passive smoking would be responsible for a thousand deaths a year. Even the most optimistic epidemiological studies estimate that the cumulative risk of death from lung cancer is one death per 1,000 people exposed to passive smoking. This risk is significantly lower than that of active smokers (in which it is in the order of 380 deaths per 1,000 smokers). However, it is decidedly uno acceptable. Recently there has been a close correlation between passive smoking and rhinopharyngitis with children's purulent otitis. The children of smokers meet much more frequently than others (38% more). In addition to respiratory diseases to passive smoking, there is also an increased risk for coronary heart disease and heart attacks of 20% (mainly due to nicotine and carbon monoxide).

HISTORY OF SMOKING

The European discovery of Christopher Columbus

he was the first European to own tobacco leaves and threw them into the sea. Bartolomé de Las Casas accurately narrates, in his reduced version of the logbook, of Columbus's first voyage, what happened on the morning of Friday, October 12, 1492, when Columbus and his men, after a 71-day voyage, landed on an island called Guanahan and has since been renamed San Salvador. On the beach, naked men came to meet him and offered him "dried leaves that give off a strong smell". Columbus accepted the tobacco leaves he had them brought on board, but then, not knowing what to do with them, had them thrown into the sea. In November of that year 1492, the sailors

Rodrigo de Jerez and Luis de Torres, while in the interior of Cuba tried unnecessarily to reach the Khan del Cathay, were the first Europeans to see smoking. They reported that the natives used to roll dry leaves of a plant called "petun" into palm leaves or corn, and after lighting one end of the paper, begin to "drink smoke on the other." Rodrigo de Jerez became a skilled smoker and kept his habit on his return to his homeland. He was probably the first smoker outside the American continent, but the smoke coming out of his mouth and nose terrified his neighbors so much that he was denounced for witchcraft. In 1501 he was sentenced by the Holy Inquisition to seven years in prison. In 1498, Romano Pane, a monk who had accompanied Columbus on his second voyage in 1493, provided lengthy descriptions of smoking habits in his book "Report on the Ancient History of the Indians." He also told how

Indians sometimes inhaled smoke through Y-tubes introduced into nostrils called "tobacus. In 1499, Amerigo Vespucci noticed that American Indians also had a strange habit of chewing tobacco. They carried two containers around their necks: one containing green tobacco leaves and the other a white powder. They took some leaves, chewed them into a ball with saliva, then passed it into the white powder and finally put it back in their mouths to chew it then for a long time. In 1535, the explorer French Jacques Cartier described the smoking habit of the natives he met on the island of Montreal (Canada): "In summer they collect large quantities of grass that dry in the sun. Only men use it. They always carry it with them and when they want it, they pulverize it, turn it on at one end and then aspire so long that they fill their bodies with smoke until they get it out of their mouth and nose like a chimney. They claim that this warms them up and makes them feel good."

1800: The century of cigar

Cigars, initially smoked only by the Spaniards, despite their high cost began to be very fashionable in the nineteenth century. The best cigars were produced in Cuba (Havana), in the
13 Short history of tobacco smoking
Philippines (Manila), Brazil and Sumatra and if the English import of cigars was only 11 tons in 1826, their consumption grew so fast that only four years later imports rose to more than 110,000 tons. It is said that in the summer of 1815 the imported Kentucky tobacco piled up in a courtyard in Florence, was bathed in a sudden storm and met with ammonia fermentation. Instead of throwing it away, he tried to use this "spoiled" tobacco as a cigar

filling, finished with a natural Kentucky band. The particular taste of this "Tuscan cigar" was so successful that the contractors of the monopoly were allowed by Ferdinand III to erect in Florence in 1818 a large factory in the former monastery of St. Orsola. In the 19th century there were manufacturers in the various states of Italy, which produced, with imported tobacco and Italian (of lower quality), snuff powders, chopped from pipe and various types of cigars. The best sellers were: Virginia, with dark tobacco of the same name, 21 cm long. with straw (made in Milan or Venice), the Tuscans, with Kentuchy fermented, 16 cm long. (made in Florence or Lucca); the Neapolitans, strong, otherwise fermented, 12 cm long. (made in Naples or Cava dei Tirreni). In 1828, two students from the German University of Heidelberg, Ludwig Reimann and Wilhelm Heinrich Posselt, first isolated the alkaloid of tobacco in pure form. They called it nicotine, provided its chemical formula (C10-H14-N2) and traced a pharmacological profile, calling it a "dangerous poison", capable of "destroying life all of a sudden".

To make it easier for cigars to ignite, in 1816 the French Francois Derosne invented the first chemical matches, while in 1827 the Englishman John Walker devised the clutch ones, putting phosphorus on wooden sticks and calling them "congreves", named after Sir William Congreve, inventor of the first military rockets. In 1852 a certain Samuel Jones marketed the product as "lucifers": comfortable, but smelly, and in 1855 the Swede Lundstrom invented, the safety match, which was lit only when rubbed on a particular surface. It was not until 1912 that Diamond Co. finally patented the canned matches, making them finally practical. During the 19th century, cigarettes were invented, which in the following century led to an explosion in the worldwide spread of tobacco smoke, as it was much faster and more practical to smoke than cigars. In fact, it is presented in 1866 by Giacomo Sormanni in his "Handbook of the smoker, grower and tobacco sniffer": "the small, slender, and gentle cigarette, voluptuous as a camellia; with nothing nothing is lit, and in the least even that is not said, burns, consumes, to be tough replaced by another" and in 1891 Oscar Wilde in his "The Portrait of Dorian Gray" admirably felt: "The cigarette is the perfect example of a perfect pleasure. It is excellent and leaves you dissatisfied. What more could you want?" In fact, as early as 14 St. Citizens et al 1600 the beggars of Seville had learned to smoke tobacco of the butts of cigars collected in the street, wrapping them in pieces of paper, called papelitos, and this habit had already been spread by sailors in Russia and the East. But historically the invention of the cigarette is attributed to some Egyptian

gunners who in 1832, during the war against the Turks, had increased their rapid fire by preparing in advance the doses of gunpowder, rolling it in paper tubes.
Rewarded with a pound of tobacco and having no pipes, they used to smoke it the same method successfully used for gunpowder, wrapping the powder in paper tubes. Their brilliant idea then quickly spread among all the soldiers of the two opposing sides: both Egyptians and Turks. During the subsequent Crimean War (1853-1856) the soldiers of France, Great Britain and the Kingdom of Sardinia learned how comfortable and cheap cigarettes, "Papirossi", used by the Ottoman allies, smoked precisely "like Turks", importing them then use in Europe at the end of the war.
In 1847, Mr. Philip Morris opened a tobacco shop in London on Old Bond Street, where he sold large hand-rolled Turkish cigarettes, and in 1854 he began to produce his own cigarettes

in a factory, located in Marlborough Street, which soon became the centre of retail tobacco trade, in England and beyond. After propaganda through leaflets, on 1 January 1848 the Milanese, to produce economic damage to Austria, began the strike of smoking and the game of the lot, both under Austrian monopoly, to the cry: "Who smokes on the street, is German or spy". To counter the strike, the Austrian authorities on 3 January sent their soldiers walking around Milan with orders to smoke cigars with ostentation. They were booed by the citizens and in the scuffles that followed some Milanese were killed with sabres. This episode of violence increased hatred of the Austrian government and contributed to the outbreak of the five-day insurgency in Milan (18-22 March 1848). The Kingdom of Italy was proclaimed on 17 March 1861 and after only one year, with the law of 13 July 1862 on the privaties of salts and tobacco, already established the state monopoly on tobacco, thus bringing together in a single administration all the manufactures of the peninsula. Cigarettes were already widespread in the United States in the 1800s, a country undergoing strong economic and demographic development. In 1871, R.A. Patterson founded the "Lucky Strike" factory, a name inspired by the 1849 Gold Rush in California, and in 1874 Washington Duke with their sons, Benjamin Newton and James Buchanan, who also opened a tobacco factory in the city of Durham in North Carolina. and, by the name of their city.

In 1875, Allen & Ginter had offered a reward of 75,000 dollars for a machine capable of making cigarettes, but it was not until 1880 that 21-year-old James Albert Bonsack patented his machine, capable of packing 200 cigarettes per minute, and so did the Dukes, who in the 1881, thanks to the work of 125 Russian Jews, they had made 9,800,000 pieces of their first cigarette, the "Duke of Durham", with only two machines, in 1884 they managed to produce and sell as many as 744,000,000 cigarettes. On April 23, 1889, the five leading American cigarette companies, including Duke Sons & Company, joined the ATC, the American Tobacco Company, which soon monopolized the entire U.S. tobacco industry. The spread of tobacco smoke was intertwined over the course of the century with the birth of the first female impulses aimed at achieving social and economic equality with men. Although the first women to smoke in public were actually the Parisian prostitutes called lorettes, as they exercised at the church of "Notre Dame de Lorettes", as early as 1840 Aurore Dupin, Baroness of Dudevant, lover of Chopin and known as George Sand , was the first lady to publicly smoke cigars in high society. As far as economic claims are concerned, the world's first "feminist" strike is due to the clawers of the manifat15 A brief history of tobacco smoking in Florence. While in 1841 325 male workers and only 20 sealers (5.3%) worked in the factory, then, due to the increased demand for cigars and the reduced female wage of the time, the ratio was reversed: in 1873 out of 1145 workers there were 939 women (82%).

In 1874(8) the economic disparity led to an unprecedented event: the seals went on strike, first obtaining limited wage increases, then in 1897, reaching economic parity with the males and in 1898 finally winning the right to the Inn. At the end of the nineteenth century, although tobacco consumption had not yet reached the proportions it will achieve only in the following century thanks to the spread of cigarettes, the harmful effects of smoking on humans began to be highlighted, even if, for example, the lung cancer, which will then be the leading cause of mortality among smokers, was still considered, an extremely rare disease, which accounted for only 1% of autopically diagnosed malignant tumours(26). On 17 January 1858, Prof. Salvatore Cacopardo at a conference in Palermo "On the health effects of tobacco use and its cultivation" marked the harmful effects of smoking on the brain, stomach, heart, nose, smell, taste and lungs: "flaccid in those such that sungella with death the faith in the cigar." He called the spread of smoking "tabacomania" and warned of the danger of habituation: "Man finds himself a slave to a habit... that makes him more than weak sensations" and the extreme difficulty in quitting: "facilitates what to prevent ree habits, very difficult to stop them". Similarly in Florence in 1869, Alfonso Baldi, in a reading on "The Tobacco" pointed to the deadly dangers of the plant: "Nicotine is such a poison that it can be, without exaggeration, compared to Prussian acid", he pointed out the various harmful effects exerted on both workers involved in the production, who on cigar and cigarette smokers, concluding that in every form "tobacco always produces the same accidents to which it keeps behind death". Despite these rare, prophetic medical warnings about the risks of tobacco, in reality the official position of medicine towards smoking at the end of the nineteenth century may well be represented by the famous "Merck's Manual", still today a reference text for physicians of the whole world, which, in its first edition, published in 1899, far from signalling the dangerousness of nicotine, indeed recommended the use of tobacco smoke for the treatment of asthma and bronchitis.

1900/1950: il boom delle sigarette

Un aneddoto storico collega l'ascesa del fumo nel nuovo secolo con la fine dell'età vittoriana. Si racconta infatti che a Buckingham Palace il 22 gennaio 1901, il nuovo re d'Inghilterra Edoardo VII, ormai sessantenne figlio della regina Vittoria, salita al trono nel lontano 1837 e da sempre nemica del fumo, entrò con un sigaro acceso in mano nel salotto ove erano raccolti gli amici ed annunciò la successione dicendo semplicemente: "Signori, potete fumare." La sigaretta è comunque l'assoluta protagonista dell'esplosiva diffusione del fumo di tabacco nel XX° secolo, infatti mentre ad inizio secolo le vendite mondiali di tabacco erano rappresentate principalmente dai sigari, con 6 miliardi di pezzi venduti contro solo 3,5 miliardi di sigarette 16 S. Cittadini et al (36%), alla fine del 1900 le sigarette assorbono da sole il 93% del consumo di tabacco nel mondo, mentre sigari e pipa restano riservati solo a pochi affezionati, e mentre nel 1889 negli Stati

Uniti erano stati venduti solo 2,4 miliardi di sigarette, già nel 1929 se ne produssero ben 122,4 miliardi. Questo boom di vendite trasformò ovviamente l'industria del tabacco in un vero impero economico mondiale. Nel 1901 nacque, per fusione, in Inghilterra la Imperial Tobacco, con sede a Bristol e nello stesso anno Duke, che già controllava il 90% del fumo americano, incorporò la Continental Tobacco e la sua società, dopo nuove fusioni, nel 1904 tornò al vecchio nome di ATC (American Tobacco Company). Per non combattersi, le due compagnie decisero nel 1902 di restare ognuna nel proprio paese d'origine e di unirsi in una società mista, la British American Tobacco Company (BAT), per tutelare interessi comuni. Nel 1905 l'ATC acquistò la compagnia Lucky Strike di Patterson e nel 1907 anche il marchio Pall Mall. Ma nel 1911 la Suprema Corte degli Stati Uniti condannò la ATC, che ormai controllava il 92% del commercio mondiale di tabacco, per violazione dello Sherman Antitrust Act promulgato nel 1890, e la costrinse a dividersi di nuovo in quattro società: American Tobacco Co. (37%), la Liggett & Myers Tobacco Co. (28%), la R.J. Reynolds (20%) e la Lorillard (15%). Per ritagliarsi più ampie fette di mercato la RJR di Reynold introdusse nel 1913 le sigarette Camel, dopo una campagna durata mesi con lo slogan "Camels are coming". Nel 1917 il nuovo prodotto ottenne il 33% del mercato e nel 1923 ben il 45%. Il loro successo era dovuto sia al gusto particolare dato dall'aggiunta di un 10% di tabacco turco, sia al prezzo di lancio: pacchetto da 20 sigarette a soli 10 cents, anziché 15. La concorrenza corse ai ripari, lanciando sigarette dal gusto simile: le Lucky Strike della ATC ("It's toasted") e le Chesterfield della Liggett & Myers ("They do satisfy"). Durante il primo conflitto mondiale (1914- 1918), si ebbe un boom del consumo di sigarette e la produzione triplicò tra il 1914 ed il 1919. Il generale americano John Pershing chiese tonnellate di sigarette: "Cosa serve per vincere la guerra? Tanto tabacco quanto proiettili". Nel 1918 l'intera produzione "Bull Durham" fu venduta all'esercito e girò lo slogan: "Quando i nostri ragazzi l'accendono, i nemici si spengono!". La disastrosa conseguenza fu che, in pratica, un'intera generazione tornò dalla guerra con l'abitudine di fumare sigarette. Nel frattempo anche le donne iniziarono a fumare apertamente, ampliando così il mercato dei consumatori. Proprio per le donne, l'inglese Philip Morris lanciò nel 1924, col motto "Dolce come maggio", la sigaretta Marlboro (dall'indirizzo della loro iniziale manifattura londinese di Marlborough Street) che aveva allora un'estremità rossa per nascondere i segni del rossetto. Già agli inizi del novecento si era compreso che il fumo di sigaretta era capace di indurre dipendenza, ma come scriveva nel 1923 Italo Svevo in "La coscienza di Zeno": "giacché mi fa male non fumerò mai più, ma prima voglio farlo per l'ultima volta. Accesi una sigaretta e mi sentii 17 Breve storia del fumo di tabacco subito liberato dall'inquietudine. Le mie giornate finirono con l'essere piene di sigarette e di propositi di non fumare più". Ma se il personaggio di Svevo doveva ricorrere alla psicanalisi per cercare di smettere di fumare, lo stesso Sigmund Freud, accanito fumatore, scriveva: "Sto meglio quando riesco a smettere di fumare, ma sono meno felice. Sento un'oppressione dello stato d'animo, in cui ho immagini di morte e vedo scene d'addio che si sostituiscono alle più abituali fantasie". Egli morirà nel 1939 per un carcinoma del mascellare diagnosticato nel 1923 e più volte trattato. Nel 1914 lo scienziato Thomas Alva Edison scrisse in una lettera ad Henry Ford che l'effetto nocivo delle sigarette era dovuto all'acroleina emessa da "l'involucro di carta che brucia" dando un'irreversibile "violenta azione sui centri nervosi, producendo una degenerazione delle cellule cerebrali, che è più rapida nei ragazzi", concludendo "...io non assumo coloro che fumano." Quasi in risposta, nel 1916 lo stesso Henry Ford pubblicò un opuscolo contro la sigaretta dal titolo "Il processo contro la piccola schiavista bianca". A rendere ancor più facile ed immediato il fumo delle sigarette nel 1932 George G. Blaisdell iniziò a produrre su vasta scala, in una fabbrica di Bradford, in Pennsylvania, accendini a prova di vento, e chiamò il modello Zippo, perché comodo e veloce come l'apertura lampo, inventata anche essa da poco tempo. Il passaggio dal sigaro alle più comode sigarette comportò un aumento vertiginoso del numero dei fumatori e della quantità individuale di tabacco fumato, moltiplicando le patologie indotte dal fumo. Il dottor Alton

Ochsner, che aveva visto un solo paziente con cancro del polmone in 17 anni di carriera, nel 1919 ne vide otto casi in 6 mesi: tutti fumatori reduci dal fronte. Nel 1912 Isaac Adler suggerì la correlazione tra fumo e cancro del polmone e nello stesso anno il chirurgo inglese Hugh Morriston Davies eseguì la prima lobectomia per cancro, anche se il suo paziente morì solo otto giorni dopo l'intervento. Nel 1914 negli Stati Uniti furono diagnosticati solo 371 casi di cancro polmonare, ma nel 1930 se ne evidenziarono 2.357 e 7.121 nel 1940, parallelamente il relativo tasso di mortalità per 100.000 abitanti passò da 0,6 nel 1914, a 1,7 nel 1925 ed a 3,8 nel 1930. Ma anche di fronte a dati numerici così allarmanti, la scienza rimase inizialmente divisa ed indecisa. Nel 1929 sulla "American Review of Tuberculosis" Frederick Hoffman, esperto statistico, scriveva "non c'è evidenza definitiva che l'abitudine di fumare sia una concausa diretta di neoplasie polmonari maligne". Peraltro, in quello stesso anno, Fritz Lickint in un lavoro pubblicato a Dresda e basato su una serie di soggetti fumatori affetti da cancro, stabilì per la prima volta con evidenza statistica un rapporto diretto tra fumo e cancro, confermato anche dalla incidenza di cancro al polmone 4-5 volte maggiore negli uomini, rispetto alle donne, che fumavano meno. Al tempo anche le riviste mediche contenevano pubblicità di sigarette. Nel 1933 la sigaretta Chesterfield fu reclamizzata sulla riviste mediche "New York State Journal of Medicine", e JAMA con lo slogan: "Pura come l'acqua che bevi ... e praticamente non toccata da mani umane". Nel 18 S. Cittadini et al 1943 la Philip Morris fece pubblicare sul "National Medical Journal" il seguente consiglio per i medici: "Non fumare è un consiglio duro da digerire per i suoi pazienti. Suggerisca invece: "Fumi una Philip Morris". È stato dimostrato che la tosse di 3 fumatori su 4 migliora passando a Philip Morris. Perché non controlla da solo i risultati?" Ma i medici, all'epoca per lo più forti fumatori, furono utilizzati addirittura come veicoli pubblicitari dalla RJR che, tra il 1946 ed il 1952 pubblicizzò così le sue sigarette: "Secondo un recente sondaggio nazionale: più medici fumano Camels rispetto alle altre sigarette! La maggior parte dei medici di famiglia, chirurghi, otorinolaringoiatri e specialisti in ogni branca della medicina ... per un totale di 113.597 medici intervistati … in tre gruppi di ricerca indipendenti ... alla domanda: "Che sigarette fuma?" ha risposto Camel. Vedi, anche i medici fumano per piacere. Il sapore pieno Camel è di richiamo per il loro, come per il tuo gusto … la meravigliosa dolcezza Camel significa tanto per la loro gola, come per la tua. La prossima volta, scegli Camel!". JAMA bandì la pubblicità di sigarette dalle sue pagine solo nel 1953 ed il British Medical Journal nel 1958. Ma al di là delle ingannevoli pubblicità, la realtà era sotto gli occhi di tutti e si cominciarono a moltiplicare gli articoli scientifici sui numerosi effetti nocivi del fumo. Nel 1939 Franz Muller in "Cattivo uso del tabacco e cancro polmonare" scriveva: "l'aumento del consumo di tabacco è la singola, più importante causa dell'aumento della incidenza del cancro polmonare" e nello stesso anno, Fritz Lickint pubblicò "Tabacco e organismo", un volume di 1100 pagine in cui incolpava il tabacco per tutti i carcinomi ad insorgenza lungo quella che lui definiva Rauchstrasse, la strada del fumo, dal labbro al polmone, ed indicava anche i rischi derivanti dal semplice fumo passivo. Nel 1938 Raymond Pearl pubblicò la sua ricerca su "Fumo di tabacco e longevità" in cui affermò che "il fumo crea un ostacolo alla longevità … proporzionale alla quantità abituale di tabacco usata", infatti: su 6.813 soggetti studiati, egli aveva riscontrato che il 67% dei non fumatori viveva oltre 60 anni, mentre tale percentuale scendeva al 62% per i fumatori moderati ed al 46% per quelli forti. Nel 1945 il dottor Roth della Mayo Clinic pubblicava “Gli effetti del tabacco sul sistema cardio-vascolare”, in cui concludeva attribuendo ai fumatori un rischio triplo di malattia cardiaca. I regimi totalitari della prima metà del novecento non potevano certo favorire la diffusione del fumo di tabacco, il cui monopolio era già praticamente in mano di Stati Uniti ed Inghilterra, e lo descrissero come un sordido vizio plutocratico. Per il Nazionalsocialismo, il mito di una razza ariana superiore fisicamente e moralmente alle altre, mal si accordava con l’abitudine di fumare e pertanto, nel quadro dell’igiene razziale, il regime promosse campagne anti-fumo ed emise precetti in tal senso rivolti innanzi tutto alla gioventù hitleriana. Inoltre nel 1939 fu proibito ai militari di fumare nelle strade e durante le marce e nel 1943 ai minori di 18 anni di fumare in pubblico. Alla fine della dittatura, la popolazione tedesca tornò poi volentieri a fumare liberamente. Anche il regime fascista osteggiò il fumo, specie tra bambini e donne, allo scopo di migliorare, fisicamente e moralmente "la stirpe nazionale". I nemici del regime, in primis ebrei e comunisti, erano infatti in genere rappresentati di aspetto sordido, con barba lunga e sigaretta in bocca. Nel 1925 si proibì il fumo sui mezzi pubblici ed ai minori di 16 anni il fumo in pubblico, infine il Regio Decreto 2316 del 1934 vietò la vendita di tabacco ai minori di 16 anni. Nel contempo si lanciavano però campagne per incrementare un'autarchica produzione di tabacco e si distribuivano gratuitamente sigarette Milit alle truppe. Durante la seconda guerra mondiale, le sigarette americane iniziarono ad essere popolari anche in Europa e ad essere preferite a quelle locali dal gusto più aspro. Dopo il conflitto, restarono con le truppe d'occupazione, ed il loro consumo aumentò, diffondendosi, come una moda, tra gli abitanti di tutta l'Europa. Dopo la guerra il cinema americano, è stato un potente mezzo di diffusione del fumo nella popolazione come portatore di un'immagine fortemente positi19 Breve storia del fumo di tabacco va del fumatore, sia maschile, che femminile: uomini, virili, maturi e sicuri del fatto loro che fumano con donne fumatrici e pertanto decise, libere, interessanti e sensuali. Il messaggio trasmesso in tutto il mondo da quelle immagini era chiaro: il fumo non rappresenta solo un piacere personale, ma anche il mezzo per mostrare agli altri una personalità che, in fondo forse, non si ha: fumo negli occhi appunto. Nella seconda metà del secolo, invece l'immagine del fumatore è andata progressivamente cambiando e nel cinema, specie in quello americano, il personaggio positivo, il buono, non fuma mai, mentre chi fuma o è il cattivo, l'assassino, o ha comunque qualcosa da nascondere, od almeno un passato difficile od un destino infausto.

1951/2000: War on smoking

It was in 1950, significantly between the two mid-century, that three important epidemiological studies were published that demonstrated the close causal relationship between lung cancer and tobacco smoke. Levin, Goldstein and Gerhardt published a work in JAMA that showed that smokers were at least twice as likely to get lung cancer(16), and in the same journal, Wynder and Graham reported that out of 684 lung cancer patients As many as 96.5% were smokers (27), while in the British Medical Journal, Doll and Hill statistically attributed to heavy smokers a 50 times higher chance of lung cancer than non-smokers(10). As early as 1930, Benson &

Hedges had launched Parliament, a type of cigarette that, to retain tobacco pieces, had a mouthpiece and the first commercial filter, consisting of a small cotton swab wet in caustic soda, and in 1936 B&W he had presented his Viceroy, equipped with a cellulose filter, believed to be capable of retaining about 50% of the smoke particles. In 1950 only 2% of the cigarettes sold had the filter, then, to meet the growing concerns of the public, brands went to war to reduce tar in smoking and the percentage of cigarettes with filter sold rose to 50% as early as 1960 and reached 90% in 1980. In 1951, RJR introduced Winston cigarettes, with a filter that enhances the taste of smoking, rather than reducing its dangerousness. In this race to make better and inexpensive filters, in 1952 Lorillard launched Kent cigarettes with a "Micronite" filter that was advertised, also on the pages of JAMA, as capable of "greater protection for health, in the history of "made of a material, pure, dust-free, completely harmless, not only effective, but so safe to be used in the air filters of operating rooms". The mysterious "pure and harmless material" was actually the infamous asbesto, known carcinogen, and the company, despite knowing since 1954 that it passed from the filter in the lungs of smokers, removed it from the trade only in 1956, 4 billion cigarettes later, without ever revealing the Secret.

After 1989, at least three Lorillard employees, employed in filter processing, died of mesothelioma, and in 1990 stockbroker Peter Ierardi of Philadelphia, who also fell ill with pulmonary mesothelioma, sued Lorillard, but his parents Lawyers could not prove that the only possible cause for his illness was inhaled asbeest with Kent cigarettes. On August 31, 1995, however, for the first time, the California Court of Appeals finally sentenced Lorillard to pay a financial compensation of two million dollars to psychologist Milton Horowitz, who fell ill with mesothelioma for smoking Kent from the 1952 to 1956. The sum was not paid until 30 December 1997, to the heirs of Mr. Horowitz, who had died in 1996. It is curious to note that a multinational tobacco company has been condemned not for the damage caused by the smoking of a cigarette of its own, but for those, even greater, caused by the filter ideally intended to reduce them. Although numerous articles published in scientific journals around the world had already repeatedly reported the health risks of tobacco smoking, the general public was still at the very beginning of this threat. In December 1952, "Reader's Digest", which with seven million copies, was the most-read magazine in America, published a two-page summary of a Christian Herald article, written by Roy Norr and titled "Cancer from the Cue". For the first time, the existence of a link between smoking and lung cancer was made known to the general public. The effect was enormous: similar articles appeared in other periodicals and all smokers began to become aware of the risks, in fact the following year, for the first time in the last twenty years, the sale of cigarettes decreased. In a 1953 paper in Cancer Research, Wynder, Graham and Croninger demonstrated for the first time that cigarette tar, applied repeatedly induced tumors on the skin of laboratory mice(28) and in a later paper, published in 1957 on "Cancer", Wynder also pointed out the existence of a precise dose-effect relationship: with the higher amount of tar applied, there was a higher incidence of induced tumors(29).

On December 8, 1953, Dr. Alton Ochsner gave a lecture in New York stating, among other things, "the male population of the United States will be decimated if cigarette smoking continues to grow as in the past, without any steps being taken to remove from them the factor that produces cancer." The next day the sale of cigarettes fell sharply and the tobacco companies decided to run for cover. Just a week later, representatives of all major companies met on December 15 at the Plaza Hotel in New York, for the first time since 1939, and planned a common strategy, creating the "TIRC", Tobacco Institute Research Committee, which under the facade of a research institute was actually intended to carry out an undeclared counter-propaganda action. Among the scientific articles of the time, it is worth mentioning the study "Preliminary Report on the Mortality of Physicians and Their Smoking Habit" published in the "British Medical Yournal" in 1954 by Richard Doll and A. Bradford Hill. The authors had interviewed 34,439 British doctors in 1951 about their smoking habits and then followed them over time by controlling their illnesses and mortality(11) and even then the study concluded that many of the doctors who had read them quit smoking were likely to quit. Doll, continuing his epidemiological work, then published in 2004, also in B.M.J.: "Mortality in relation to smoking: 50 years of observations on English male doctors", concluding that 80% of non-smokers arrive at the age of 70, but only 50% of heavy smokers; 33% of non-smokers live up to 85 years, compared to only 8% of heavy smokers, while life expectancy for smokers compared to non-smokers decreased by an average of 7.5 years, rising to 10 in the case of heavy smokers(9). In 1954, Eva Cooper launched the first lawsuit against a tobacco company, holding her responsible for her husband's death from lung cancer, which she smoked. In 1957, the R.J. Reynolds Tobacco Co. was acquitted on the basis that "a fatal case of lung cancer can be developed, in such a short time, after Cooper's alleged smoking of Camel cigarettes. , under the pressure of various forms of advertising." After this precedent, for about 40 years no tobacco company lost a lawsuit, always using the same defensive strategy: choose the best lawyers without sparing expenses and make the trials last as long as possible in order to exhaust the lesser resources However, he denies that cigarettes are harmful to health, but at the same time that if smoking really hurts smokers should have known. In the mid-1990s, the situation changed dramatically because the publication of secret documents from the tobacco industry revealed the lies and fraud perpetrated against smokers and the use of class-action class-action lawsuits. and, as a result, better legal colleges, as lawyers in the United States can be paid not only with a fixed amount agreed in advance, but also through a percentage of the compensation obtained. On January 4, 1954, out of 448 American newspapers, which reached over 43 million readers, the TIRC announced its birth with an ad titled: "A sincere statement to cigarette smokers." It stated, among other things, that medical research points to numerous causes for lung cancer but there is no evidence that smoking cigarettes is one of these causes, while the statistical assertions linking cigarette smoking to the disease could in fact be applied to every other aspect of modern life; For our part, we are sure that our products are not harmful to health and in any case, as we have always done, we will always work closely with those who pursue the protection of public health. In April 1954, the TIRC published a booklet entitled "A Scientific Perspective on the Cigarette Controversy" in which 36 scientists questioned the relationship between cigarette smoking and health problems. The publication was widely circulated, because it distributed to more than 170,000 doctors and to all newspapers and radio stations in the United States. On July 26, 1954, W.C. Hueper gave a lecture in Brazil at the 6th International Cancer Congress, entitled "Lung Cancer and Environment".

Considering the text in favour of their cause, the multinationals made a pamphlet that was also distributed to newspapers, radio and 123,000 doctors. In 1950, the Federal Trade Commission found cigarette advertisements, "physical benefits" misleading, and in the same year condemned Lorillard Co. for advertising its Old Gold cigarettes as "the most low tar and nicotine content" because the figure, although technically true, referred to a difference from other cigarettes, so modest as to make the message deceptive. In 1955 he also forbade any reference to "throat, larynx, lungs, nose...or energy, digestion, nerves, or doctors" to appear in cigarette advertising. In March 1957, Reader's Digest magazine, continuing its campaign, revealed that the level of tar and nicotine in filter cigarettes had been progressively increased to the point of using unfiltered brands, and in July of the same year. year, he confirmed his statement, providing comparative data of the various cigarettes: the smoke of camels without a filter contained 31 mg of tar and 2.8 of nicotine per cigarette, while that of Winston, despite the filter, respectively 32.6 and 2.6 thanks to use of a stronger tobacco mixture. In response, the American Tobacco Co. pushed the B.B.D.O. agency that ran both its own advertising and Rider's Digest to make a choice, and, though reluctantly, the magazine was abandoned. In 1957, John A. Blatnik, chairman of a government sub-committee, submitted a report to the Federal Trade Commission, calling for its intervention against misleading advertising 22 S. Citizens et al of filter cigarettes and in 1958 the report Blatnik was brought to Congress. In it he declared, among other things: since "... Filter cigarettes provide roughly the same level of tar and nicotine as those without filter, ... the F.T.C. has failed in its institutional duty." Soon after, Blatnik was removed from the presidency and his subcommittee unceremoniously dissolved. In 1957, in the American Journal of Obstetrics and Gynecology, Winea J. Simpson gave the children of smoking mothers twice as likely as others to be born prematurely, born less and at birth or death within the first month of life(22), while in the same year the British Medical Research Council published "Tobacco smoke and lung cancer" in which it reiterated that "... The report is of direct cause and effect"(1). In 1959, in an article in JAMA, Burney confirmed this position of the British Public Health Service on the relationship between cigarettes and lung cancer, complaining that "... It still receives little public and scientific attention."

The special focus on lung cancer was linked to the sharp increase in the relative mortality rate detected in those years around the world, but particularly in the United States (29,000 deaths in 1956) and, above all, in England, where in 1952 it was Also died of lung cancer was the beloved King George VI, who had always been a heavy smoker. In fact, in those years there was an increase in malignacurities covering the whole respiratory tree(5) and in particular the larynx, as early as 1960 Ruppmann in Germany(20) and in 1963 Carfagni and Celestino(4) in Italy, had shown a correlation between increased incidence of larynx cancer and tobacco smoke. On July 27, 1962, the Surgeon General, the Surgeon General, the Head of Federal Public Health Services in the United States, Luther Terry appointed the ten members of an "Advisory Assembly on Smoking and Health", whose task was to establish, objectively and definitively, whether or not there is any damage to health from smoking cigarettes. On July 17, 1963, legal counsel Addison Yeaman wrote in a confidential memo to Brown & Williamson Tobacco Corp. "Nicotine has two types of beneficial effects: it enhances the pituitary-adrenaline response to stress and regulates body weight. In addition, nicotine is addictive. Our business is therefore to sell nicotine, an addictive pharmacological agent, effective in calming the mechanisms of stress"; The report will conclude that "it has some unattractive side effects: it causes or predisposes to lung cancer, contributes to some cardiovascular diseases and is responsible for emphysema." On January 11, 1964, a date chosen specifically on Saturday so as not to upset the stock market, the first copies of the Terry report, a 387-page work based on the analysis of more than 7000 scientific articles, were delivered to the press in a White House room. it was stated that cigarette smoking in men causes lung and larynx cancer, in women it is a probable cause of lung cancer, and is also the most important cause of chronic bronchitis, concluding that: "Smoking cigarettes is a health risk of importance in the United States as to authorize appropriate corrective action"(24).

It was only at the end of the presentation that journalists were left free to go out and access their phones. The Terry report was widely circulated around the world and generated such a reaction in public opinion that in the following days there was a 20-25% drop in cigarette sales. After the first, 31 other Reports by the Surgeon General, about one a year, were published between 1967 and 2010, which blamed smoking for other diseases. Among them: "Smoking and Heart Disease" (1967), "Smoking and Low Birth Weight" (1969), "Risks from Pipe and Cigar Smoking" (1973), "Unpaetic Tobacco Risks" (1979), "Smoking and Coronary Heart disease" (1983), "Smoking and Chronic Obstructive Bronchitis" (1984), "Consequences of Involuntary Smoking" (1986), 23 A Brief History of Tobacco Smoking "Nicotine Addiction" (1988) and "Prevention of Smoking in Young People" (1994), "Women and Smoking" (2001), "Children and Passive Smoking" (2007), "Biology and Behavioral Bases of Smoking-Related Diseases" (2010). On February 27, 1964, the American Medical Association accepted a donation of ten million dollars from six cigarette companies for tobacco research. In return, he spent ten years publishing reports on the relationship between cancer and smoking and sided with the tobacco industry, sending a letter to the F.T.C. on 28 February stating, among other things, that, since "... more than 90 million Americans use tobacco ... the economic lives of growers, producers and traders are linked to industry; and local, state, and federal governments are recipients and dependent on many millions of dollars in tax revenue."

In Italy, law No.165 of 10.4.1962 banned the advertising of smoking products and in 1965 cigarette advertising was also banned on British television while the United States Congress enacted the "Federal Decree on Cigarette Labels and Advertising. "The following warning from General Surgeon' on the side of each packet of cigarettes: "Beware: cigarette smoking can be risky to your health." In 1970 the message was amended in the most categorical: "Beware: the Surgeon General has determined that cigarette smoking is risky to your health." In accordance with the Cigarettes Smoking Act of 1969, starting at midnight on January 1, 1971, the United States banned radio and television advertising of cigarettes, with a loss of advertising revenue of more than 220 million dollars per year. In the 1960s, epidemiological and laboratory research repeatedly demonstrated a dose-effect relationship between smoking and the risk of contracting diseases. For example, the Italian Candeli in his work "Tobacco Smoke and Human Health" of 1965, recommended, to reduce the risk of lung cancer, cigarettes with "filter capable of absorbing a good percentage of nicotine" and "low tar". Finally, in 1966 a technical report to the Surgeon General concluded that "a low rate of tar and nicotine corresponds to a less harmful effect" and recommended "a progressive reduction in tar and nicotine yield in cigarette smoking". Therefore, for 30 years the scientific community and public health authorities have promoted the production and trade of light cigarettes, that is, low yield in tar and nicotine. Unfortunately, there is the phenomenon, called compensation, for which the smoker, in order to obtain the dose of nicotine that he needs, tends to inhale more deeply, to smoke more cigarettes and to the end, thus nullifying, with an increase in quantity, the reduction of Concentration. In fact, the printing of threatening package warnings, far from discouraging smokers, has in fact protected the industry from accusations of misleading advertising, while light cigarettes, thanks to compensation, have favoured sales.

In 1990, it was established in Europe that, "because the higher the tar content and the higher the risk of lung cancer", the tar content of each cigarette should drop to 15 mg. 12 mg from 1997 and the current 10 mg since 2001. Moreover, in November 2001 the "Monography 13" of the US National Cancer Institute questioned for the first time the usefulness of a reduction in tar, saying: "The evidence is not convincing that changes in the composition of cigarette from 1950 to the mid-1980s produced a significant reduction in the burden of diseases caused by cigarette use, both for smokers and for the general population"(19). In January 1967, the book "Smoking Is Safe" was published with wide publicity. The scientific facts in the dispute between smoking and health and a clear surprising conclusion." by Lloyd Mallan. In it, many of the scientists interviewed stated that smoking was not dangerous and that, if it had been, the coal filter would have ensured excellent protection. Before 24 S. Citizens et al that the year ended, the book was taken off the market for a congressional investigation into alleged funding received by the author by the tobacco industry. In January 1968, True magazine published an article by renowned sports journalist Stanley Frank entitled "Smoking or not smoking. That's still the problem," concluding that "the risks of smoking cigarettes may not be as real as we are led to believe." He then repeated the same concepts in an article in the National Enquirer titled "The link between cigarette and cancer is nonsense. 70,000,000 falsely alarmed smokers!"

Frank was actually an employee of the public relations agency that created the TIRC, and had been paid by a tobacco industry that had also been able to correct the text before publication. On January 3, 1971, Philip Morris President Joseph Cullman, interviewed on the CBS program "Front to nation," stated among other things, "I believe that it has not been proven that cigarettes are not safe." "The Surgeon General's Committee has concluded that nicotine is not a health risk ... and that cigarettes don't get addictive." 'If smokers' children have a low birth weight, that doesn't mean they're not healthy - some women may prefer to give birth to younger babies!' In 1972, an RJR researcher wrote in a confidential memo: "The tobacco industry must be considered as a specialized segment ... whose products contain and supply nicotine, a potent chemical that... Fortunately for the industry, it gives habit and has unique physiological actions ... to give satisfaction." In a Philip Morris document of the same year, which remained secret until 1988, it was written: "The cigarette should be imagined not as a product, but as a wrapper. The real product is nicotine... The cigarette is the distributor of a unitary dose of nicotine... A puff of smoke is the vehicle for nicotine... Smoking is definitely the best vehicle for nicotine and cigarette the best smoke dispenser." In a 1974 article in the Family Practice News, Dr. Feinstein, secretly paid for by the tobacco industry, had the courage to declare "the more cigarettes a person says about smoking, the more likely he is to be examined by his doctor for the risk possible lung cancer. So smoking cigarettes contributes more to the diagnosis of lung cancer than to the genesis of the disease."

In 1979, the magazine "Mother Jones", having to publish an article on smoking addiction, begged tobacco companies to refrain from advertising for that issue. In response, the companies cancelled the entire multi-year advertising contract, imitated, out of corporate solidarity, from those of liquor. In Italy, Law 584 of 11 November 1975 banned smoking in public places: hospitals, museums, cinemas, schools, theatres, libraries, waiting rooms and public transport. Law enforcement was advertised by an anti-smoking campaign that had the slogan: "Who smokes poisons you too. Tell him to stop." The tobacco industry was deeply concerned by the emergence of movements for the rights of non-smokers, as well illustrated by this secret memo of 1978: "What the smoker does to himself is his business, but what he does to the non-smoker is a matter completely Different... Let us consider this the most dangerous development so far for the very survival of the tobacco industry ... The strategic and long-term antidote to the issue of passive smoking is to develop and widely publicize a clear, credible medical proof that passive smoking is not harmful to the health of non-smokers." Instead, in January 1981 the British Medical Journal published an epidemiological study by Dr. Takeshi Hirayama that scientifically tested the risk of developing lung cancer as a result of exposure to passive smoking(15). The author had followed, patiently and meticulously, typically oriental, for 14 years about 92,000 non-smoking Japanese women divided into two groups: married to men who smoked and with non-smokers respectively. 25 A brief history of tobacco smoking Compared to tobacco (32 lung cancers out of 21,895 women), the wives of those who smoked up to

19 cigarettes a day had a 60% higher risk of dying from lung cancer (86 cases out of 44,184) and the wives of those who smoked 20 or more sigaretts and had a 90% increase in risk (56 out of 25,146).

The tobacco industry strongly challenged Hirayama's conclusions in newspapers around the world. First he was credited with miscalculations by the well-known statistician Nathan Mantel, who later beed the criticism, then emphatically reported the results of a similar work, conducted in America by Garfinkel, which had indeed found an increase in lung cancer from smoking passive, but not statistically significant(14). After 30 years, the Japanese study is still considered valid today and it is estimated that passive smoking increases the risk of developing lung cancer in non-smokers by about 30%. Repeated scientific confirmations led Surgeon General C. Everett Koop to conclude, in the 19th report of 1986, that: "Exposure to environmental tobacco smoke can cause non-smoking diseases, including lung cancer ... It is also clear that the simple separation between smokers and non-smokers in the same airspace can reduce, but not eliminate the exposure of non-smokers ... There is an increased risk of reduced lung function in children and adolescents whose parents smoke"(18). The Rose Cipollone case is the first lawsuit for damages won by a smoker against a multinational tobacco company. Mrs Rose Cipollone, of Clear Italian origin, who had started smoking cigarettes in 1942, at the age of 17, had surgery for lung cancer in 1981 of right lobectomy and the following year of right pneumectomy. In 1983, he sued the manufacturers of his favorite cigarette brands, but died of cancer in 1984 at the age of 58. The trial she filed continued, however, and in 1988 the judge found that three firms had created a conspiracy "vast in scope, convoluted in purpose and devastating in the results", and ordered the Liggett Group to pay compensation of 400,000 dollars for having provided, until 1966, false guarantees of safety on its products, unfortunately the family, for lack of funds, had been forced to abandon the case, before obtaining the payment of compensation. On the contrary, the first European lawsuit brought against a tobacco company that began in Finland in 1988 came to its conclusion thirteen years later: the supreme court ruled that the applicant Pentti Aho, who died of cancer in 1994, was solely responsible for the disease that has developed. In 1989, due to the need to comply with EEC rules, a Directive of the Council of Ministers imposed the display on cigarette packets of their nicotine and tar content and forced three sentences to be printed on the cigarette, clearly in sight for the smoker: "Smoking causes the "severely harms health," "smoking causes cardiovascular disease" and other optional phrases. These phrases, instead of being a real brake on tobacco consumption, were, in fact, the necessary premise in order to be able to hold the smokers themselves responsible for any conscious damage they suffered, while providing an alibi for the harm they have suffered. multinationals of smoking enriched with the proceeds from the sale of cigarettes, which these pathologies had caused. Meanwhile, the Environmental Protection Agency (EPA) continued its fight against passive smoking in 1993 in a 510-page report entitled "Respiratory Effects of Passive Smoking on Health: Lung Cancer and Other Diseases" declared cigarette smoking Class-A carcinogen and in 1994 the Federal Pro-Children Act was enacted that prohibited smoking in any public indoor facility used as a school, place of care or library for children under 18. In the same year, McDonald's banned smoking in its 11,000 restaurants, and the state of Mississippi was the first to sue the tobacco industry in order to cover up health care costs incurred to treat smoking-related diseases. The journalist Jacob Sullum, sharply criticized in an article in the "Wall Street Journal" the conclusions of the EPA and the hindu S. Citizens et al stria of tobacco paid him 5,000 dollars and 10,000 reason magazine for which he worked, to republish the article at full page on all the major newspapers for a few days, accompanying it with the slogan "If we had said it, you might not believe it". So the public saw more criticism of the EPA report than the report itself.

The 20th Report by the Surgeon General in 1988 was devoted to 'nicotine dependence'(6) and to clarify once and for all the existence of this drug-effect of cigarette smoking and whether tobacco multinationals were aware of this, on 14 April 1994, the Managers of 7 tobacco companies (RJR, Liggett, US Tobacco, Lorillard Tobacco, Philip Morris, American Tobacco and Brown & Williamson) were called to testify before the U.S. Congress on nicotine addiction. All seven managers, before the sub-committee chaired by Henry A. Waxman, swore that nicotine was not addictive. In August 1995 Jeffrey Wigand, former chief researcher of Brown & Williamson, recorded an interview for the TV show "60 Minutes" in which he stated that Sandefur, the president of his firm, had lied to Congress and that even the tobacco industry it enhanced the effect of nicotine, accelerating its absorption from the lungs through the use of ammonia. CBS blocked the broadcast and partially aired it only six months later. In 1993, he died of lung cancer at the age of 47. Peter Castano, a smoker from the age of 16, and his widow Diane, determined to get compensation from the tobacco industry, turned to a lawyer who recommended a class action lawsuit and in February 1995 a staff of 60 lawyers was ready to involve 90 million smokers. In March 1996, Liggett accepted an economic agreement which, among other things, agreed to devote 5% of its profits to anti-smoking campaigns for 25 years, but two months later, in May 1996, the Court of Appeal ruled that the class-action was ineligible, both for the excessive number of members, than because of the legislative differences between the various states involved. After the agreement reached in 1997 between the tobacco industry and Mississippi to compensate with 14.7 billion dollars the medical costs incurred to treat smoking diseases, other states took the same path and in November 1998 the multinationals of the Tobacco preferred to sign a federal agreement with 46 states, called the Master Settlement Agreement.

Under it, strict advertising restrictions were put in place to limit smoking among young people, and the industry was committed to a huge compensation of 206 billion dollars, even if it was delayed over 25 years. In 1998, Brown & Williamson, the producer of Lucky Strike, was ordered to pay a total of 750,000 dollars to Grady Carter, a smoker with adeno-lung cancer, and a further 550,000 dollars in compensatory damages and 450,000 dollars for punitive damages to the family of Roland Maddox, who died of lung cancer. In 1999, Philip Morris was ordered to pay Patricia Henley, who had lung cancer, with a million and a half dollars in compensatory damages and a further 25 million in punitive damages, then reduced to 9 million on appeal. On March 23, 2005, the Supreme Court rejected further appeals and forced Philip Morris to pay Mrs. Henley 10.5 million in damages, in addition to 6.2 million accrued interest. In 1998, the class-action lawsuit by pediatrician Howard Engle, a heavy smoker since his youth and ill with emphysema, also began. In July 1999, the Florida court convicted the tobacco industry of "fraud, misrepresentation, negligence, concealment, conspiracy" and in April 2000 three smokers were awarded a total of 13 million dollars for representative use: Frank Amodeo, who had larynx cancer, Mary Farnan and Angie Della Vecchia, who had lung cancer. Finally, in July 2000, punitive damages of astronomical magnitude were established, the largest ever imposed in the world: 145 billion dollars! If confirmed, the tobacco industry would have risked bankruptcy, but in May 2003 the 27th Short History of Tobacco Smoking in Florida overturned the verdict, ruling the plaintiffs' group too disparate and the Florida Supreme Court decertified the class-action, admitting only individual cases.

21st century: The new millennium Today scientific knowledge on the damage caused by smoking in those who consume cigarettes and passively breathes smoke has brought obvious changes in behavior throughout the Western world: no more smoking in the premises public, shops, cinemas, trains, planes, while initiatives, medical and commercial, aimed at helping to stop smoking are increasing. The percentage of smokers, male and female, is steadily decreasing, cigarette advertising is now banned and tobacco multinationals have already suffered enormous economic damage for all the convictions suffered in the trials that have been concluded and further heavy damages are expected in the coming years. Surgeon General Regina Benjamin, in her last report on smoking in 2010, concludes by saying: "The time to act decisively and firmly to end one of the deadliest epidemics our country has ever known, is now." But, at the world level, the situation is quite different. 6.3 trillion cigarettes have been produced worldwide, or more than 900 cigarettes for each of the Earth's nearly 7 billion inhabitants, man, woman, or child(21). In addition, between 1970 and 2000, while tobacco consumption in Western countries fell slightly from 2.3 million tonnes to 2.1 million tonnes, it almost tripled in the same period, from 2 million tonnes to 5.3 million tonnes. , bringing the world total to increase from 4.3 million tonnes to 7.4 million tonnes. China alone produces 35% of all cigarettes in the world and consumes 31% of them(13).

It is estimated that around one billion men are currently smokers worldwide, of which 311 million are Chinese (about 60% of the male population), while 131 million are Indians: the emerging CINDIA alone expresses almost half of smokers worldwide(21). The so-called "smoking epidemic" (see Figure 1) develops in each country through four successive phases(17) lasting twenty, thirty years each: it starts with a progressive increase in the percentage of smokers first only among males (stage 1), then also among women (stage 2), then begins a reduction limited first to males (stage 3), and then also extended to women (stage 4), while the harmful effects have a staggered trend of about 50 years, with a mortality curve that reaches the maximum for the men in stage 3 and women in stage 4. Today (see Figure 1), Western countries are in phase 4 of the epidemic, while the eastern countries have just entered phase 2(12) and that is why the WHO predicts, according to the model already lived in the West, that the epidemic produced by smoking will kill a number of from the current 5.4 million per year to 10 million per year in 2030 and more than 80% of them to developing countries(25). Dr Margaret Chan, Director-General of the

WHO, said in 2008 that "reversing this totally predictable epidemic must now be considered a top priority for public health and for political leaders in every country in the world"(25), to To prevent tobacco smoke from writing yet another dark pages in its already very long history in the coming years.

CONCLUSIONS

Smokers are the best consumers in theworld: faithful, hardened, constant, indifferent to the consequences. For years with all weather, in any place, in any condition I am able to find a tobacconin and a few euros to smoke. Smoking is a very well thought out mechanism, replicated and replicable to most consumption, to the many induced needs, as useless as it can create dependence, physical and mental, to shape our image and fill our time.

Although cigarette smoking causes about 5 million premature deaths worldwide each year, the percentage of smokers who manage to complete a disadmortation protocol is still very low. The World Health Organization – given the enormous health and economic impact of smoking and its clinical consequences – has tried over the years to promote, at different levels, strategies for smoking cessation. Mass information campaigns, increased tobacco taxes, the spread of easily accessible psychotherapeutic protocols and drug therapies, have been the workhorses proposed in recent decades. Among the various methods, pharmacotherapy was certainly the most effective, but also the most expensive, thus remaining accessible exclusively to a selected user. The low accessibility of pharmacotherapy and the increasing incidence of smoking in the most socio-economically disadvantaged groups has therefore prompted various experts in the field to identify alternative therapeutic strategies. In this context, the use of natural extracts such as Cytisine was included.

Don't wait any longer.... Stop smoking and you'll be happier!

Contrary to those who are convinced that quitting smoking the quality of their life can get worse, those who have done so now say they are more serene and healthy. Quitting smoking requires a great willpower, but the effort has paid off well: those who have done so now feel that they are happier, more serene and even healthier. To the devil, therefore, the fear that saying goodbye to cigarettes can be a tragic decision that can worsen the quality of one's life. On the face of it it may seem that you may lose something, but after that you find that you have earned a lot.

Take back your life !!

Disclaimer

This book is not intended as a substitute for the medical advice of physicians. The reader should regularly consult a physician in matters relating to his/her health and particularly with respect to any symptoms that may require diagnosis or medical attention.
(health, quit smoking)

Made in the USA
Middletown, DE
07 July 2021